Copyright © 2018 Alena Knezevic
All rights reserved.
ISBN-13: 978-1721140893

MY FIRST DENTAL ENCYCLOPEDIA

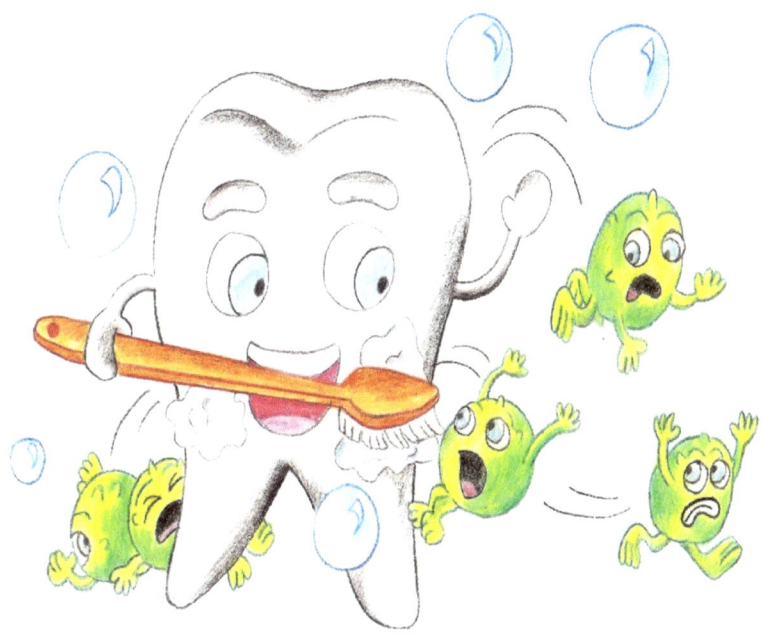

Written by Alena Knezevic DMD, MS, PhD

Illustrated by Rina Risnawati

Explore the dental world through this children's dental encyclopedia!
My First Dental Encyclopedia will help parents and children to learn about teeth, how to keep them clean and healthy.

Special thanks to our amazing Cheryl J. Park, DDS FACP, for taking time editing this book.

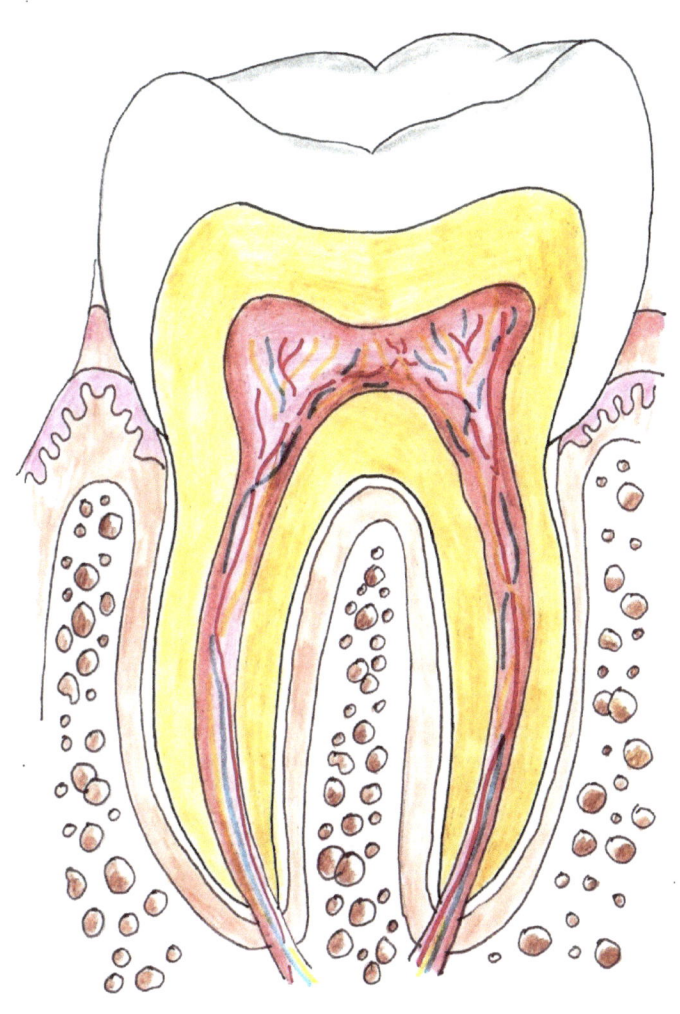

Tooth – is the hardest substance in human's body.

How do the teeth look like?

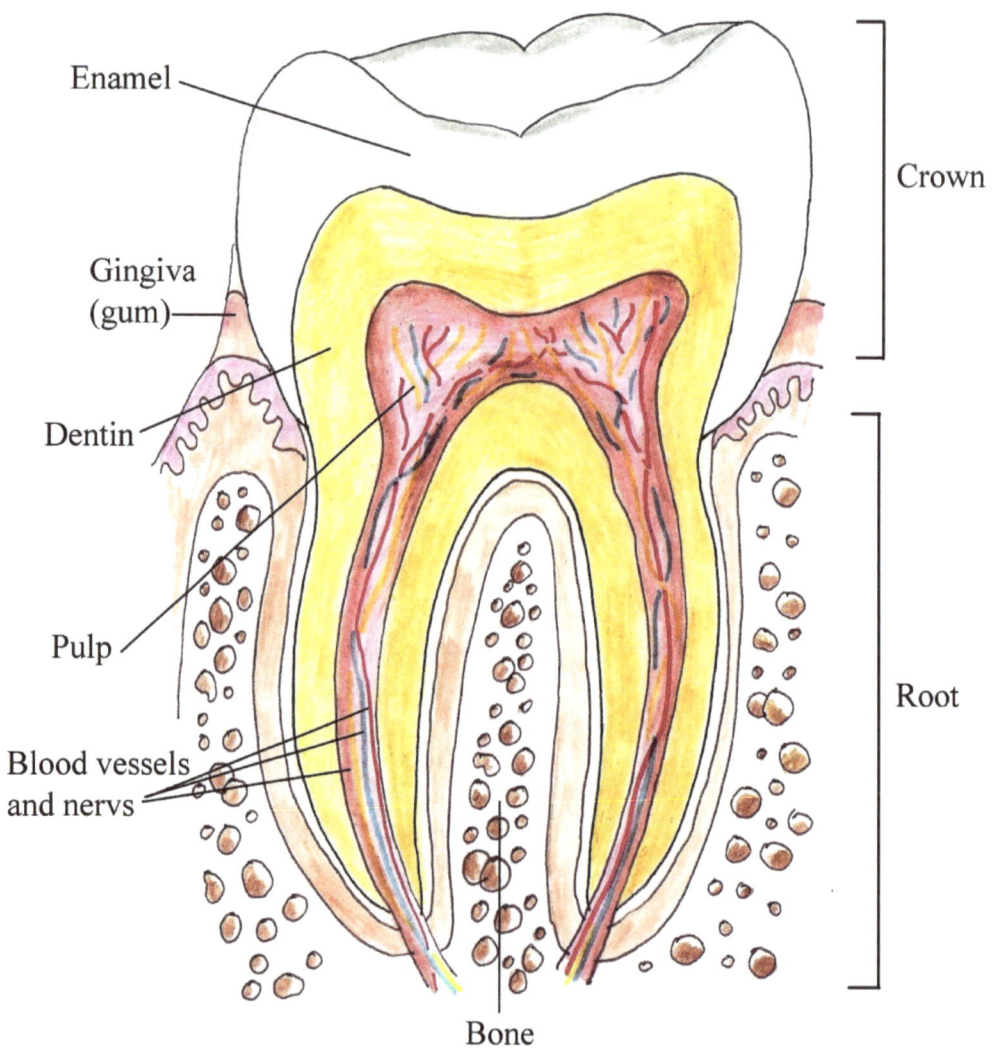

Tooth has a crown and a root. Crown is made of the outer layer – enamel and inner layer – dentin. In the inner part of the crown and root is dental pulp which is made of blood vessels and nerves and shortly said, it gives the tooth its life.

The teeth which are covered with lips are called front or anterior teeth, incisors and canines, while the teeth covered with cheeks are called distal, back or posterior teeth, molars and premolars.

The frontal teeth look like a shovel ...

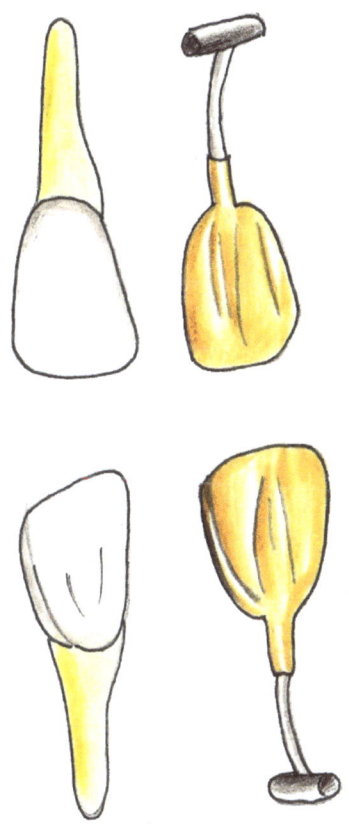

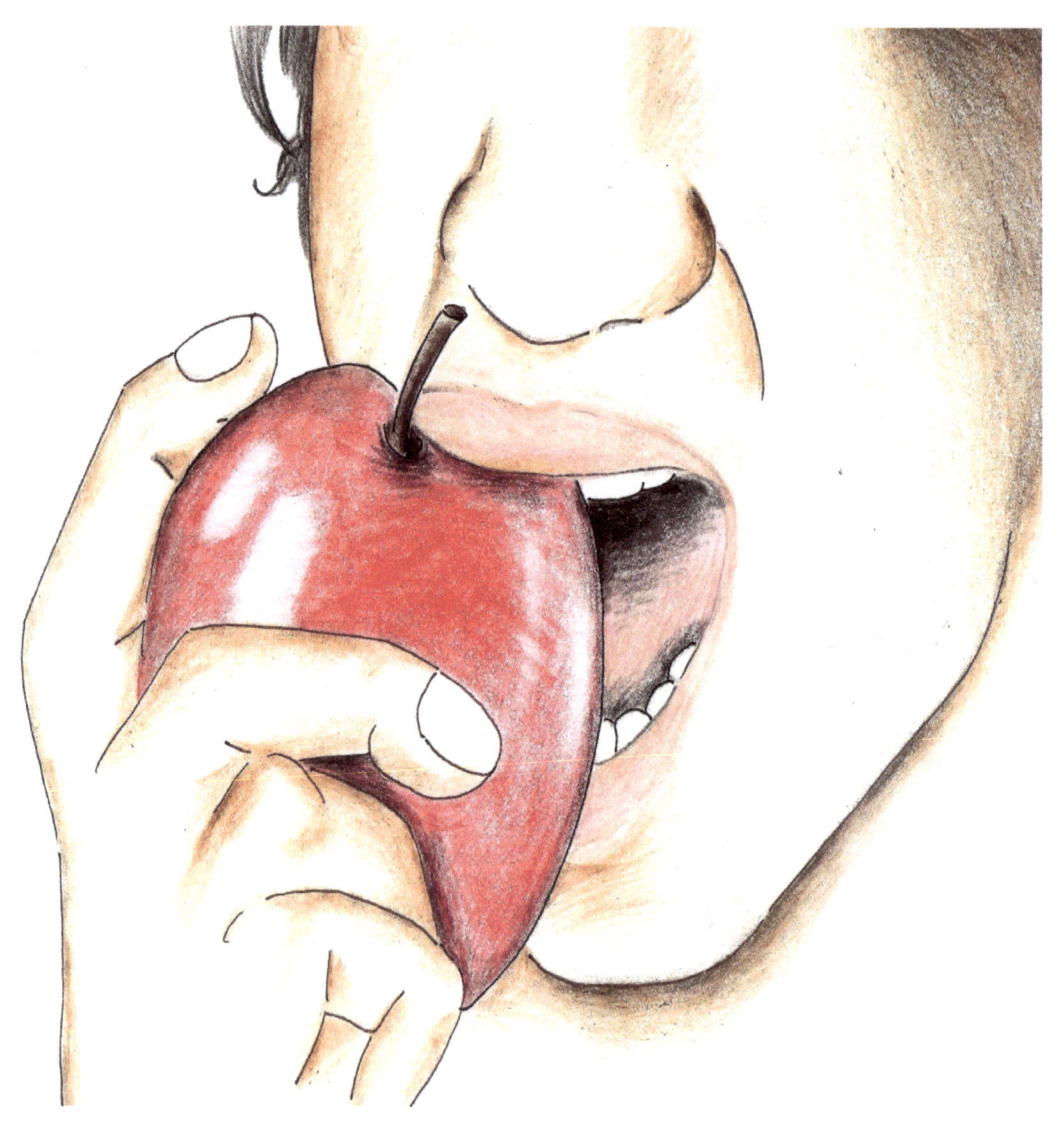

…. and they are used for cutting the food.

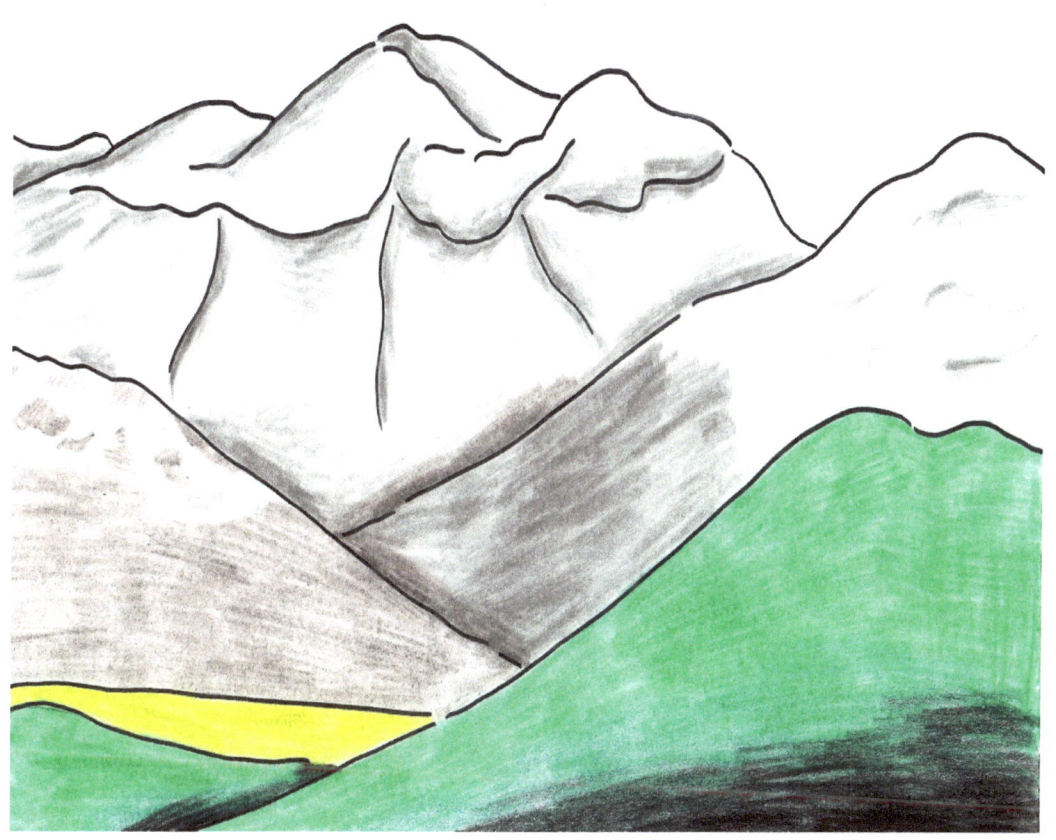

The distal teeth look like mountains and valley, they are not flat, they have cusps and fissures.

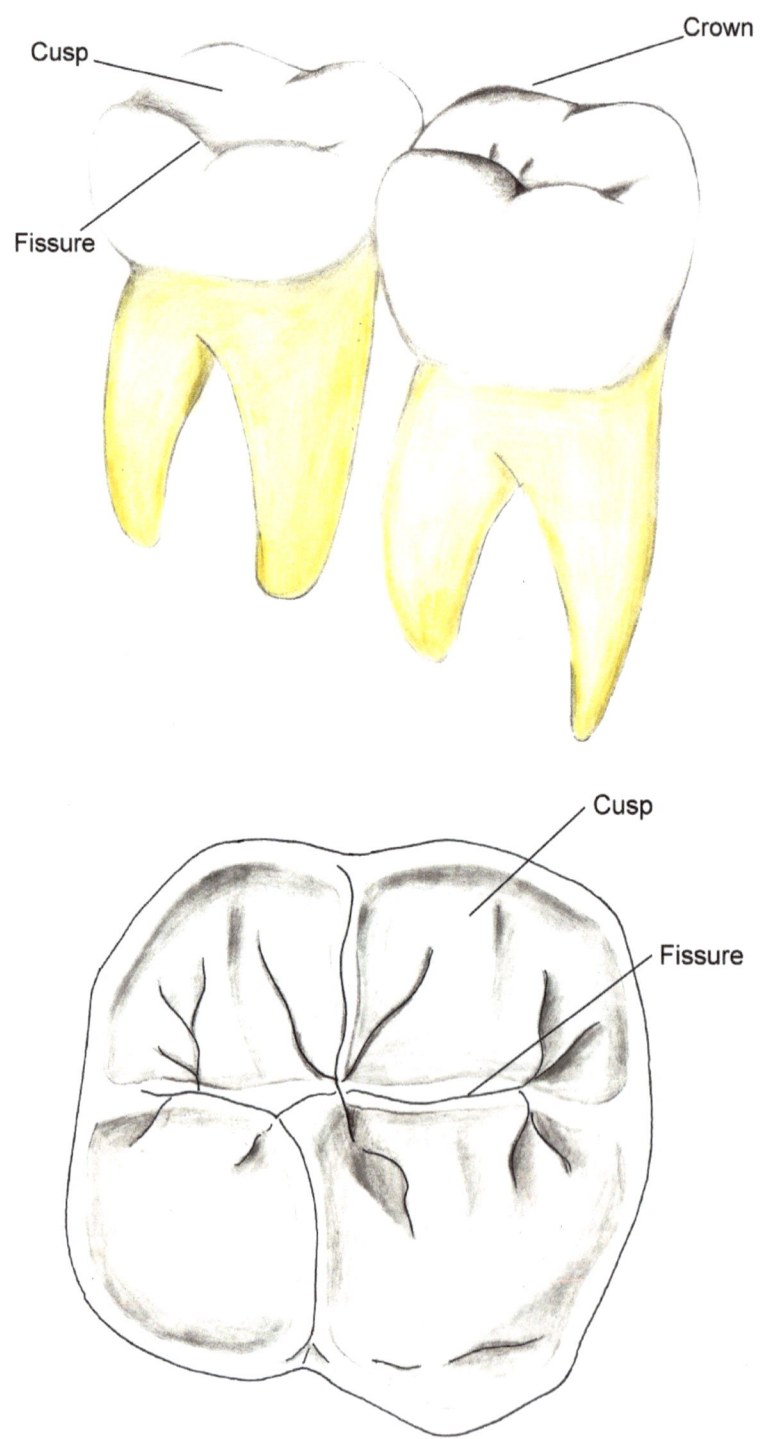

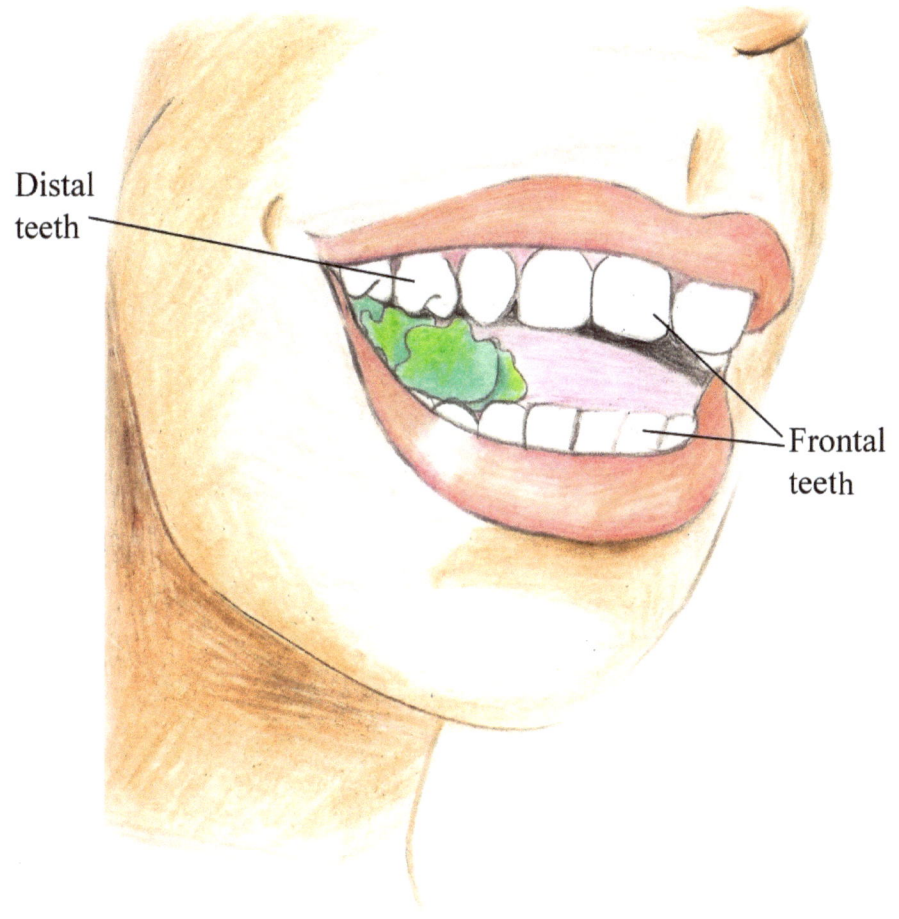

The molar and premolar teeth are used for grinding and chewing the food.

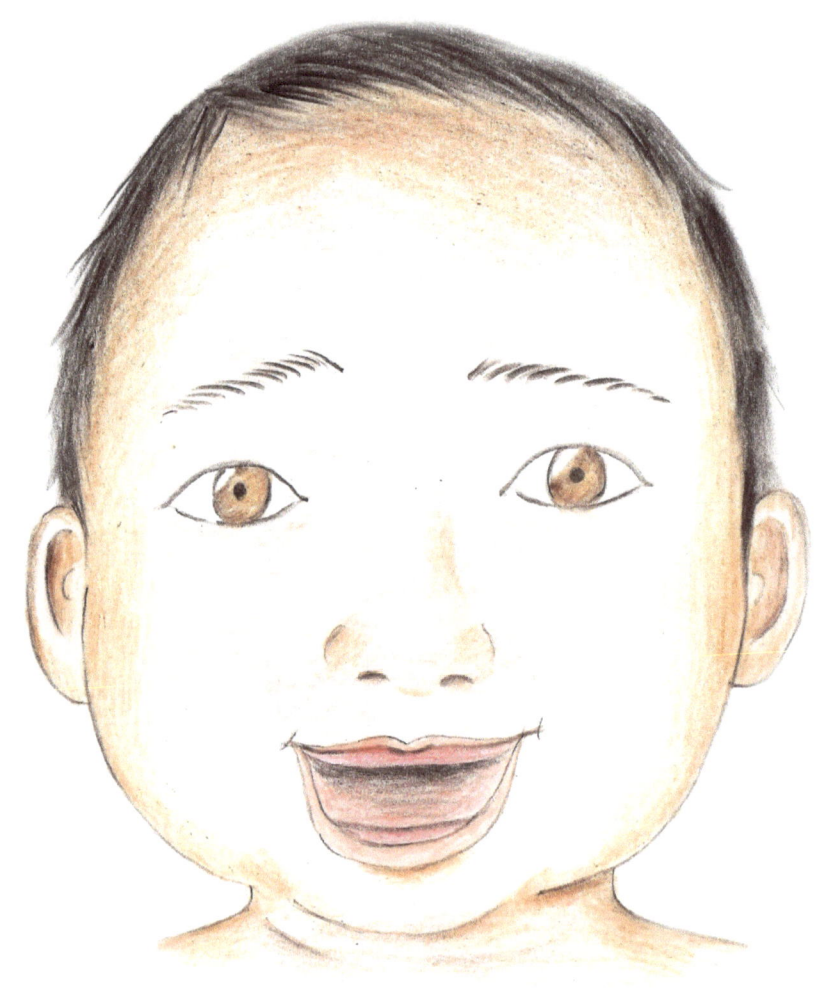

Usually, newborns do not have teeth ...

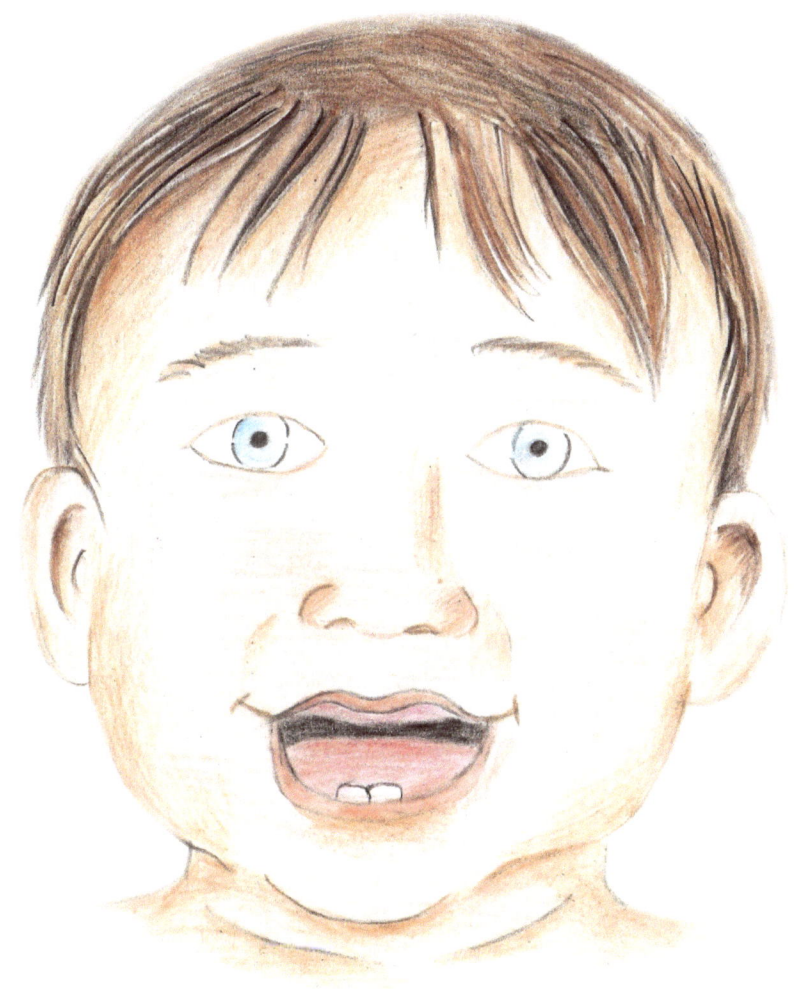

... but some babies are already born with teeth.

At 6 months of age a baby starts getting teeth, one by one ... and by the end of the second year you should have all teeth in your mouth – total of 20; 10 in the lower jaw and 10 in the upper jaw. Let's count together: 1, 2, 3, 4, 5, 6 ... 20.

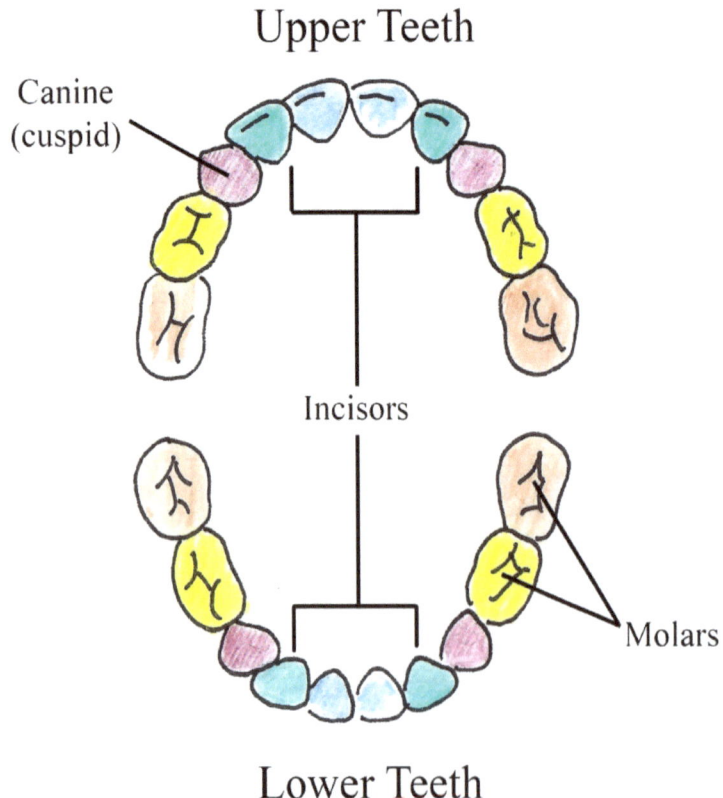

Deciduous (baby) teeth

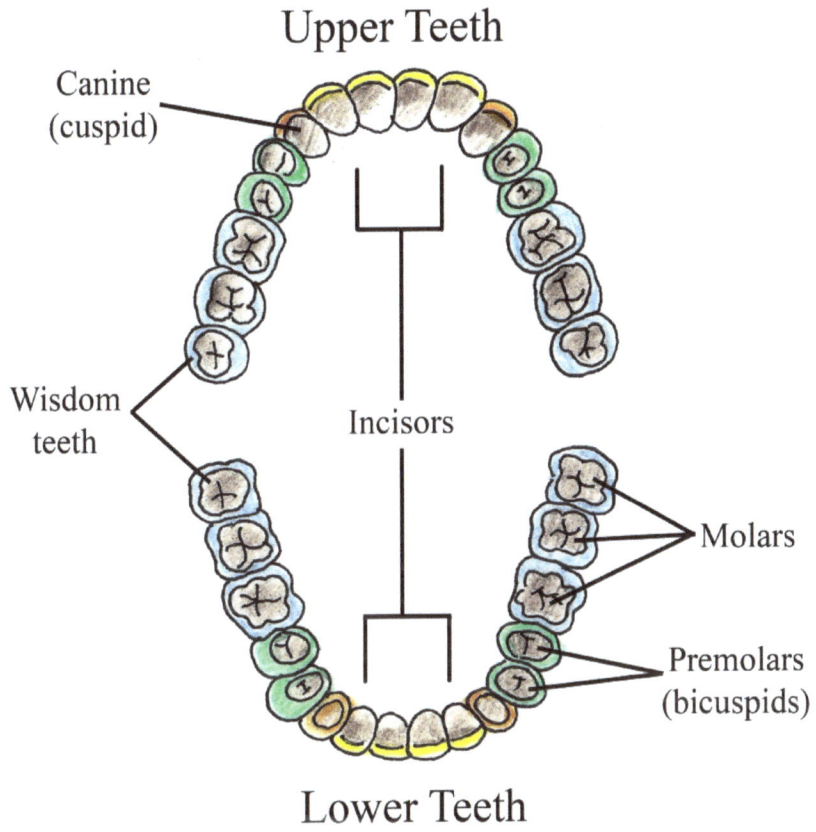

Permanent teeth

Baby's teeth are called deciduous teeth and they will start to fall out as you reaches six years. Thereafter, you will start to get permanent teeth, total of 32; 16 in the upper jaw and 16 in the lower jaw. Let's count again: 1, 2, 3, 4, 5, 6 ....32. If you take care of them you should have them for all your life.

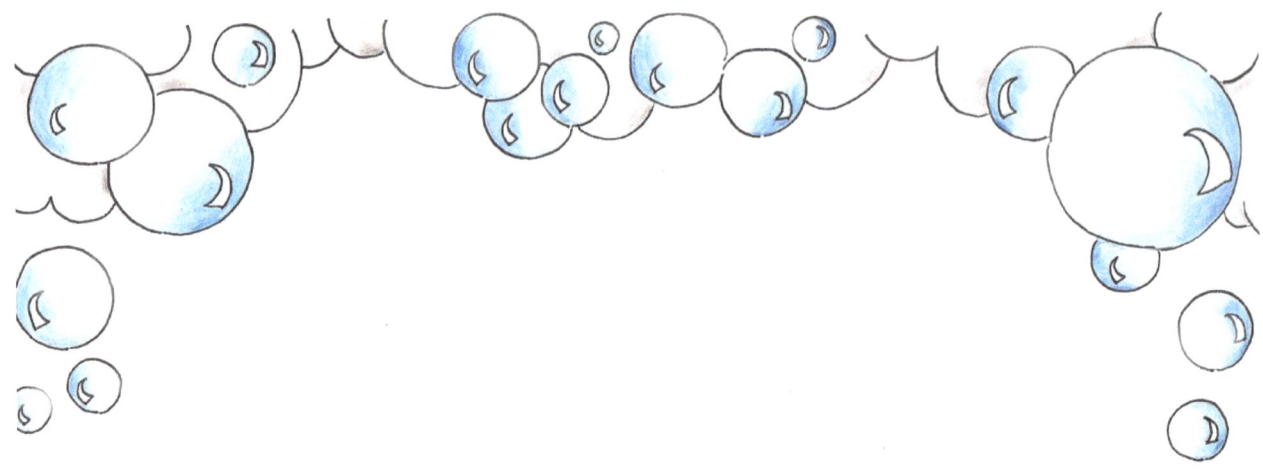

To keep your teeth **healthy, you** should brush them properly and frequently and watch what you are eating.

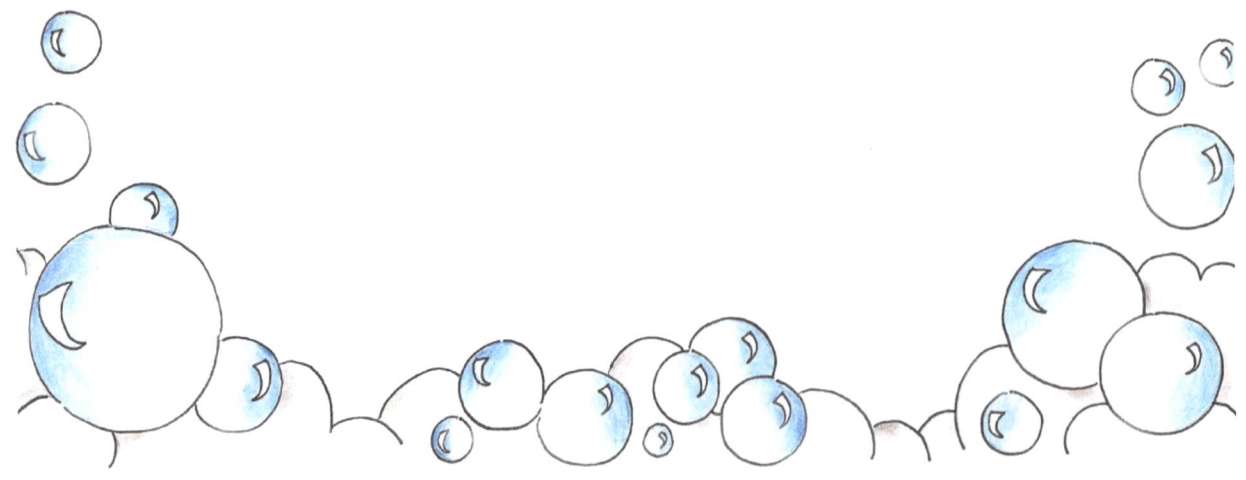

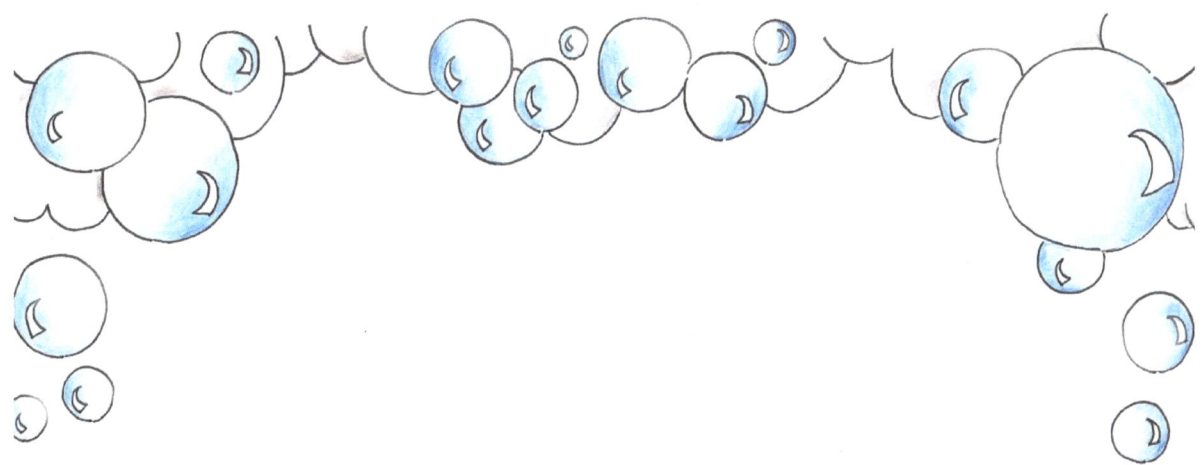

What do you eat in order to keep your teeth healthy?

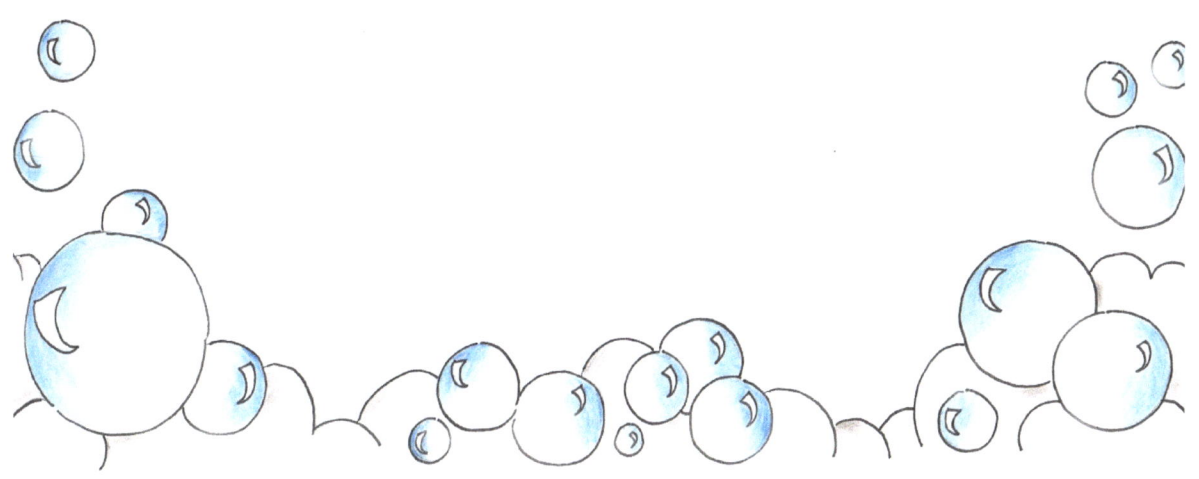

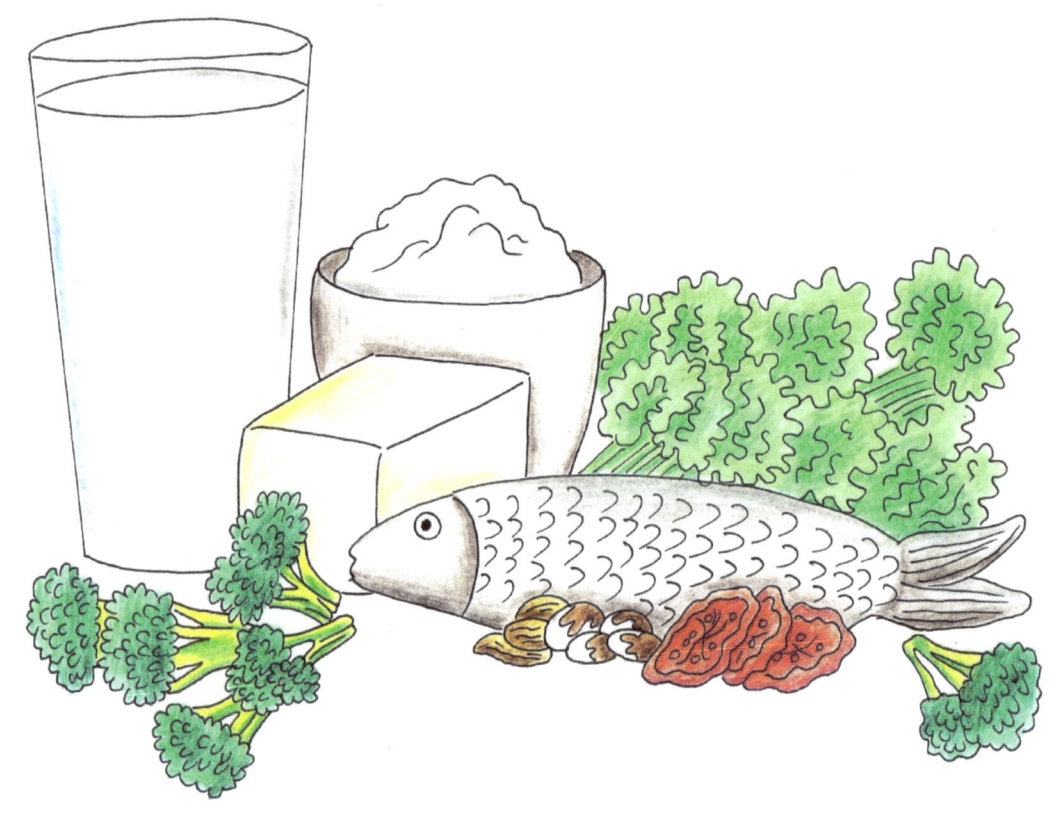

Dairy products such as milk, yogurt, cheese, as well as kale, green collard, mustard greens, turnip, spinach, broccoli, sun dried tomatoes, fish, almonds, Brazilian nuts, and dried beans - are good sources of calcium, which keeps your teeth strong and healthy.

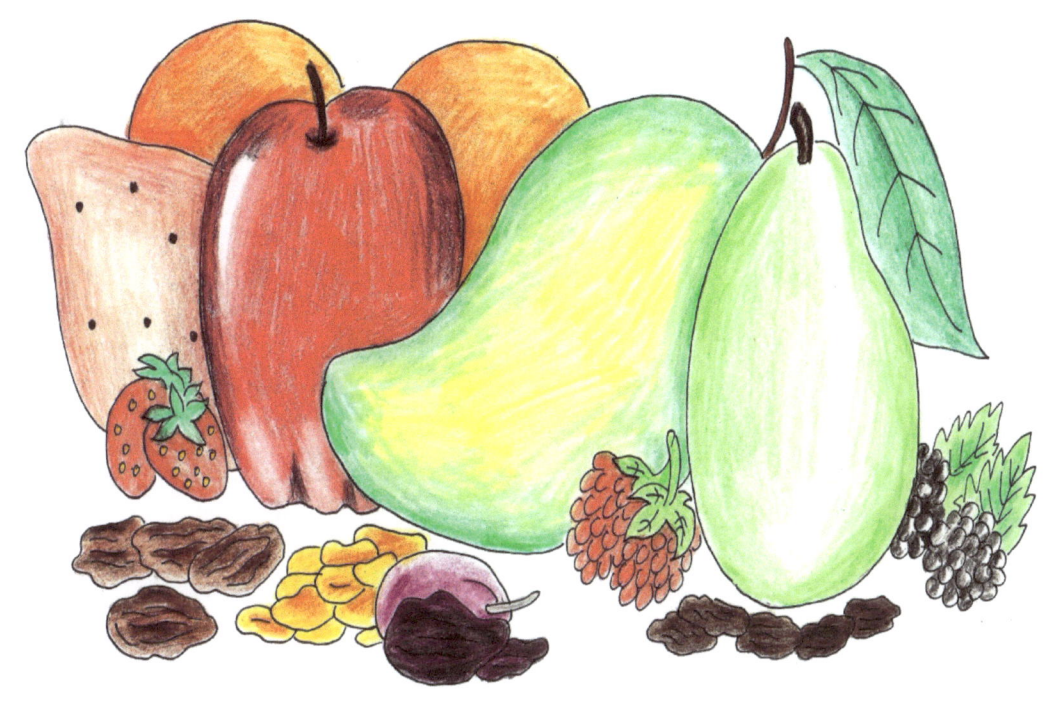

Fruits (mangos, pears, prunes, apples, raspberries, strawberries, blackberries, oranges), dried fruits (dates, apricots, raisins and figs), veggies (avocados, sweet potatoes, artichoke, spinach, carrots, sweet corn, brussels sprouts), and legumes (beans, lentils, peas), peanuts, almonds and bran, are rich in fiber which will keep saliva flowing and help create mineral defense against tooth caries (cavities or decay).

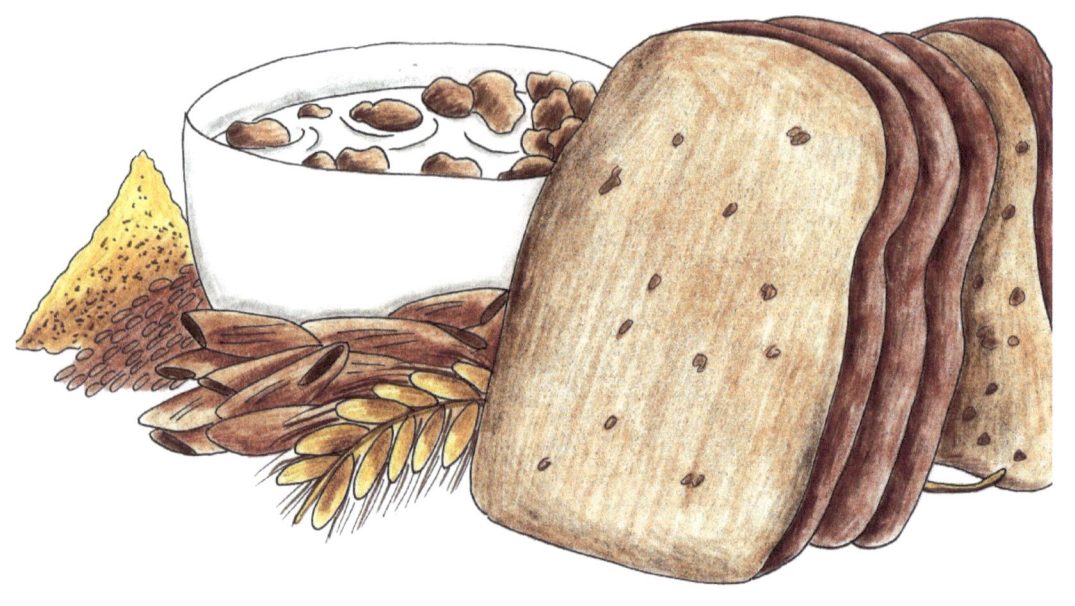

Whole grains are also high in fiber and provide B vitamins and iron, which help keep gingiva healthy. Further, they provide magnesium - very important ingredient for healthy bones and healthy teeth. Foods such as bran, brown rice, whole-grain cereals, millet, quinoa, bulgur, whole grain corn (corn meal), whole grain pasta and whole grain bread are excellent sources of whole grains.

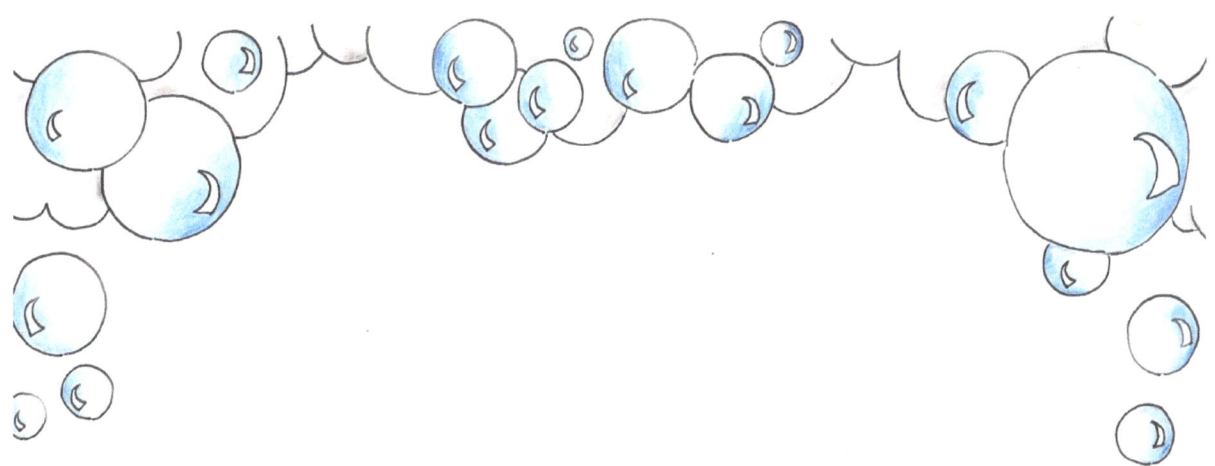

And of course, do not forget vitamins! *Vitamin A* you can get from dark greens or yellow fruits and vegetables, from eggs and dairy products. In different kind of fruits, you can find a plenty of *vitamin C* while *vitamin D* you will get from egg yolks, fatty fishes and dairy products.

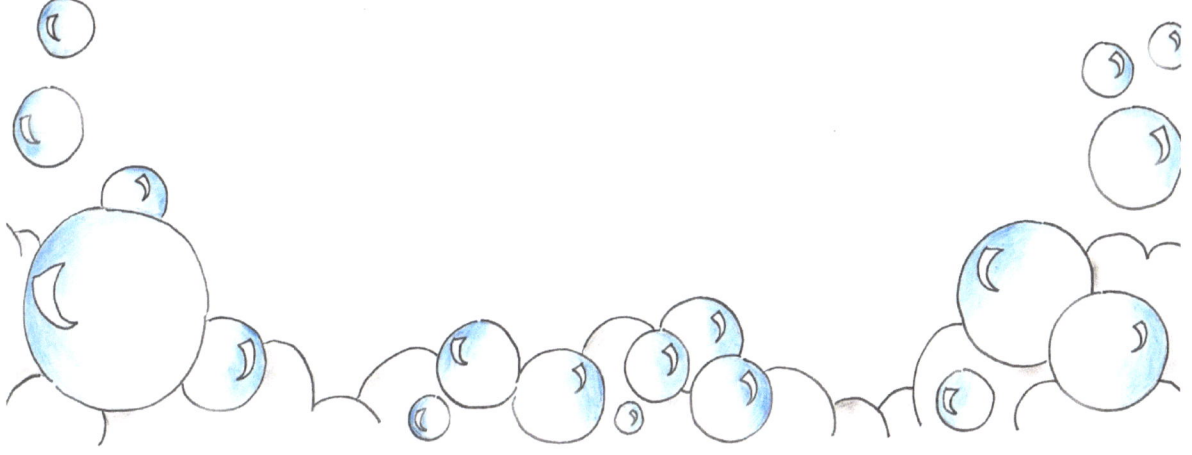

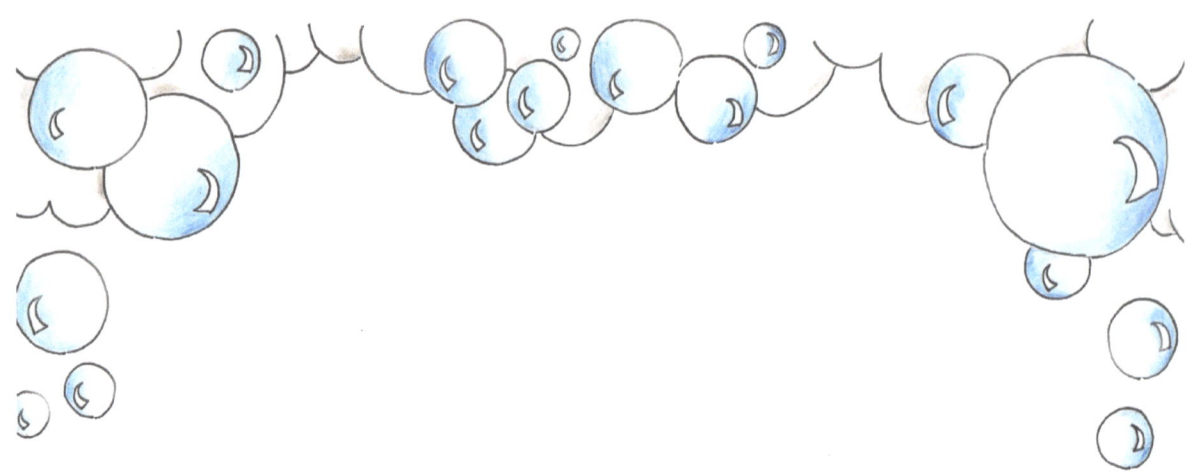

*F*ocus on choosing healthy foods. Try to keep away from sweets as much as possible, because sugar coupled with plaque (bacteria and food debris left in the mouth) have a tendency to weaken tooth enamel, leaving your teeth susceptible to tooth caries.

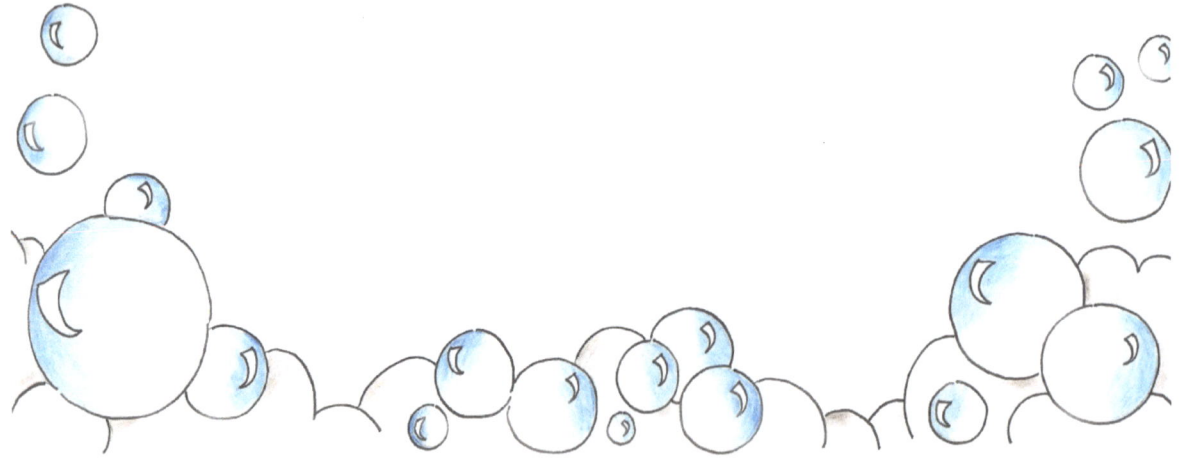

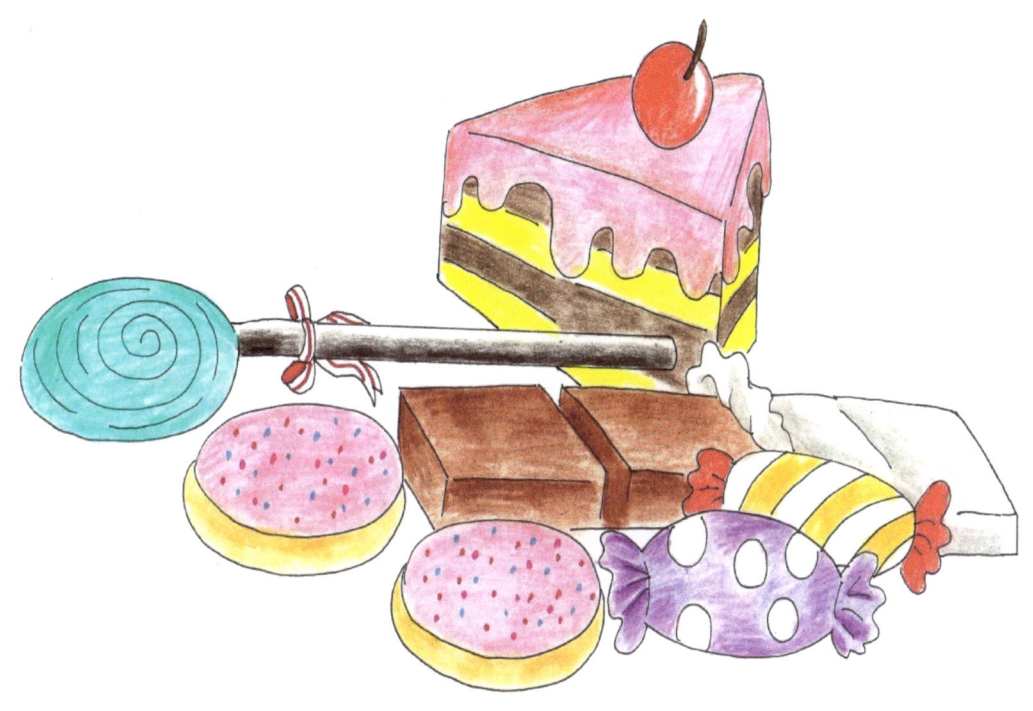

Therefore, avoid sweets like candies, lollipops, chocolate, sugar cookies ... and take healthy snacks like apples, dried fruits and carrots while reading or watching TV.

In short, when we are talking about healthy diet that is good for your teeth and your whole body, try to follow the rules of the food pyramid.

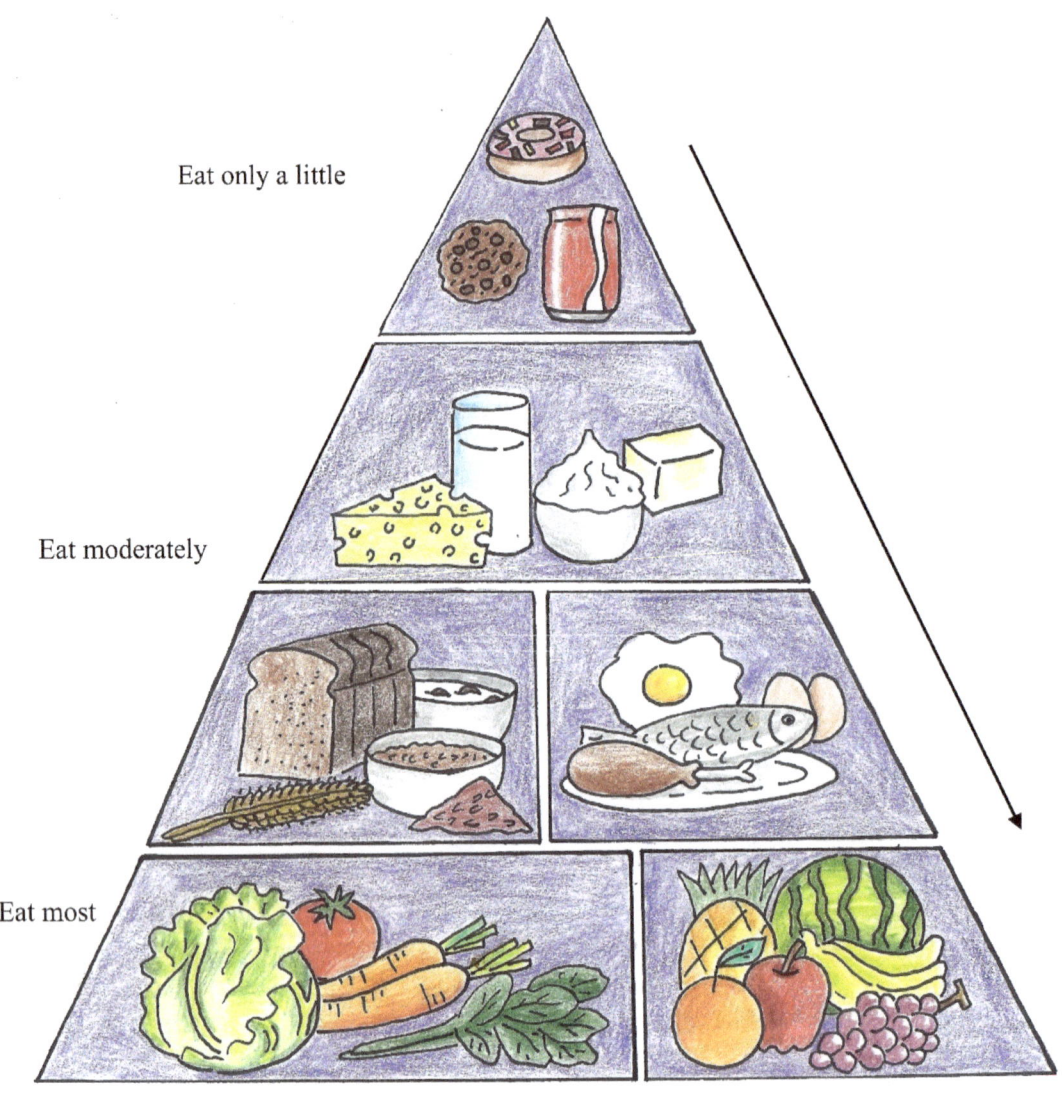

The food pyramid is structured to show you a healthy serving of all the necessary food groups you need throughout the day.

When we were talking about sugary snacks we mentioned plaque and tooth caries.

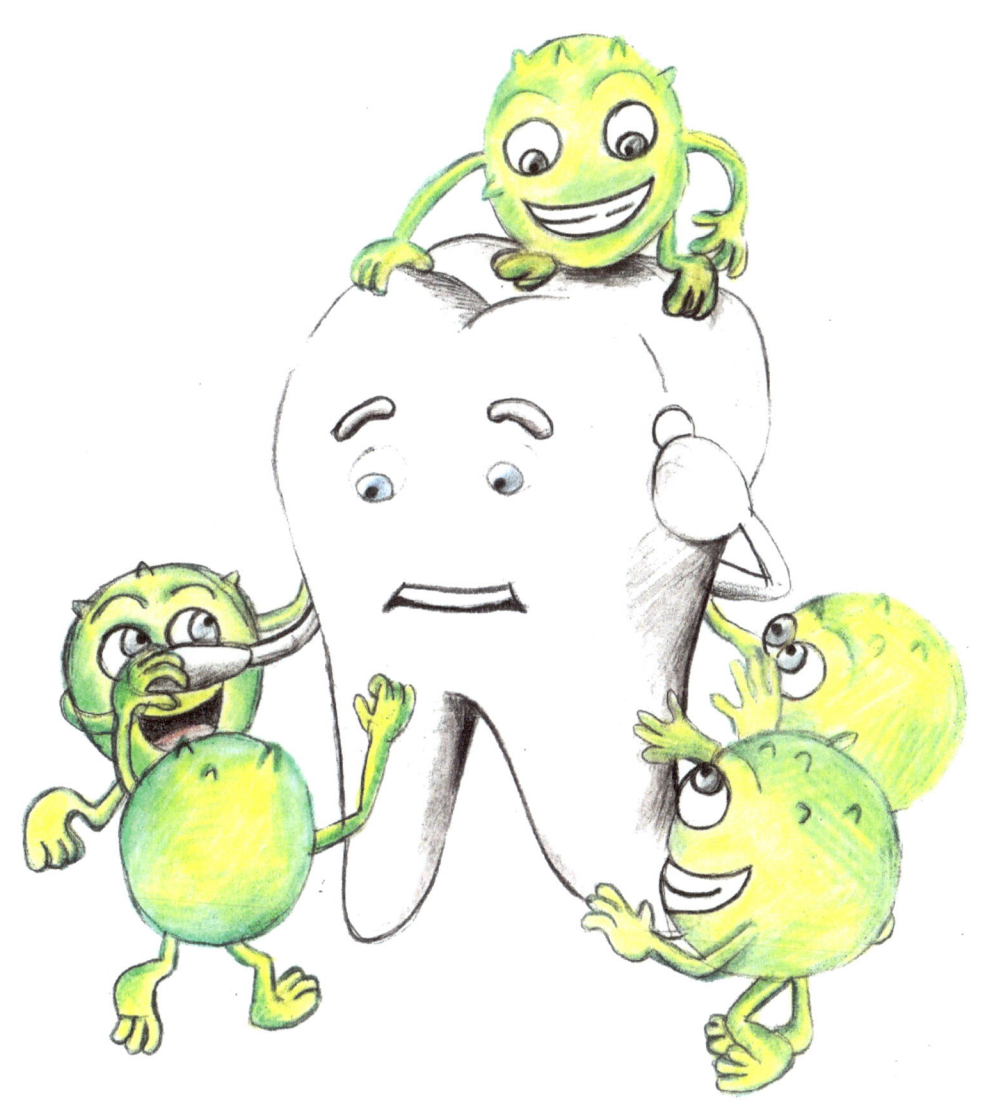

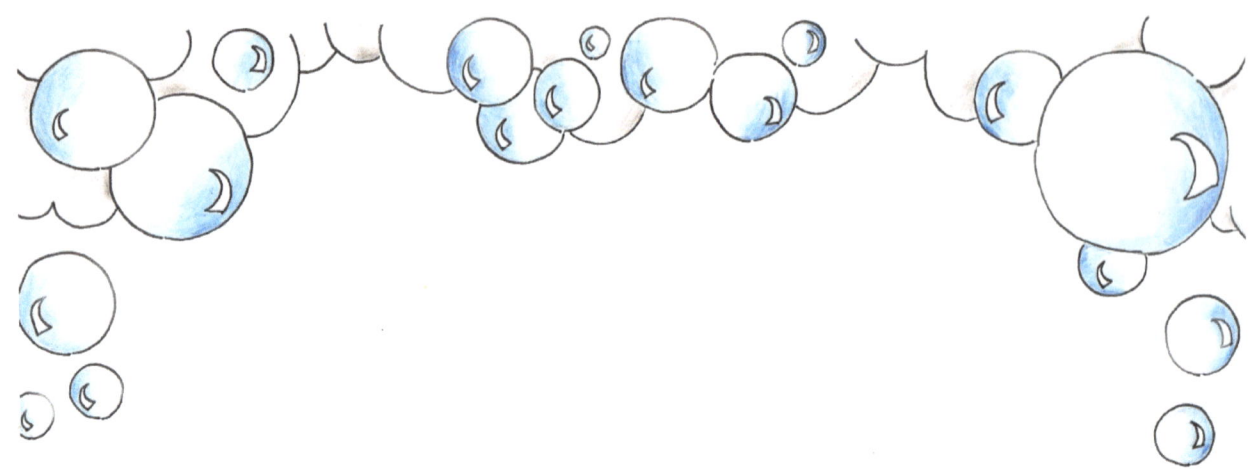

So, what is plaque?

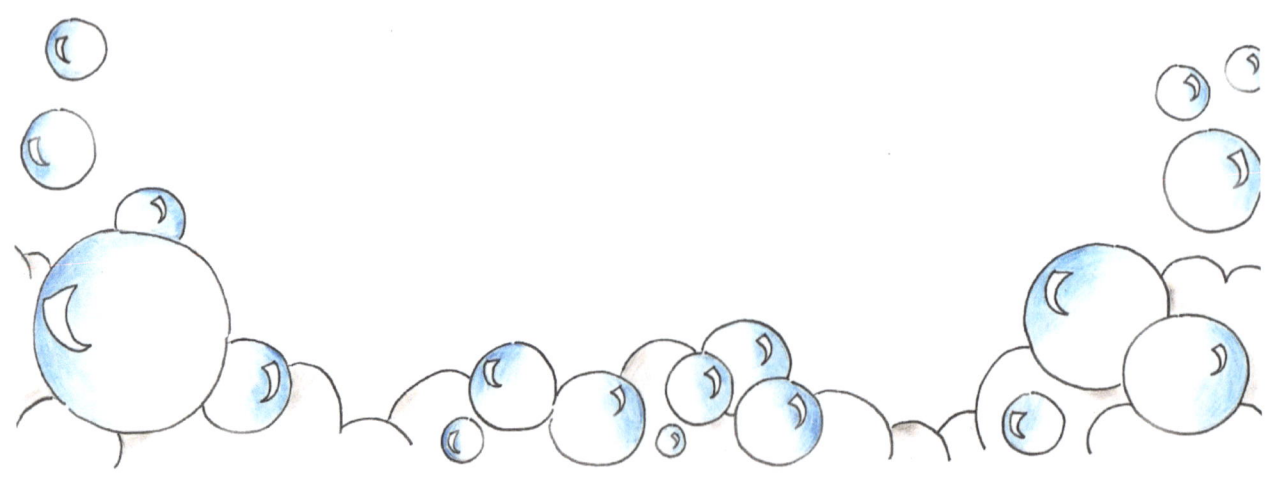

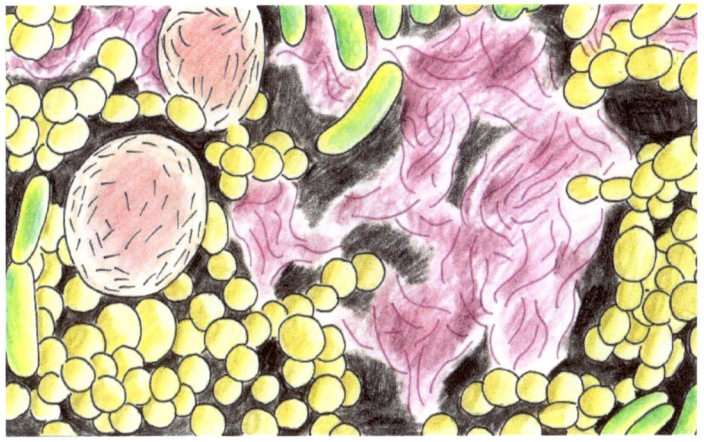
Bacteria

Plaque is a cluster of live and dead small microorganisms, bacteria, and food residue on a tooth surface left after improper tooth cleaning or not cleaning at all.

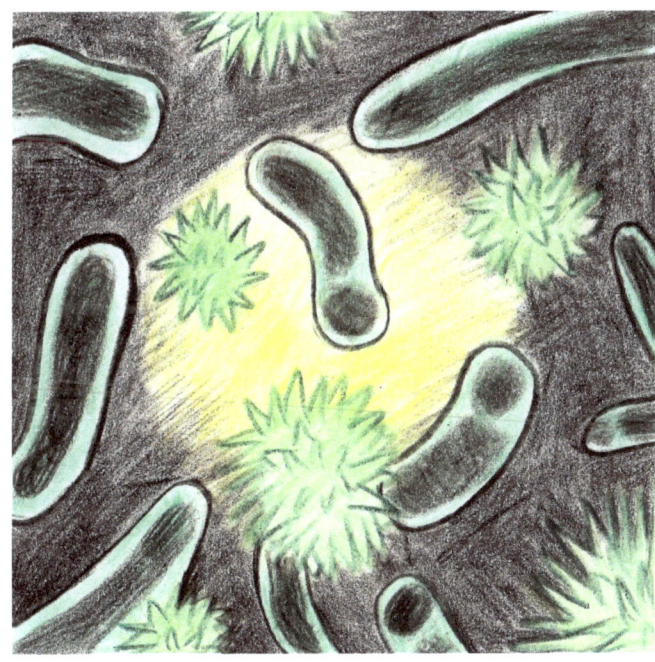
Bacteria

It is usually a pale yellow color and when it is still soft it can be removed with a toothbrush and a toothpaste.

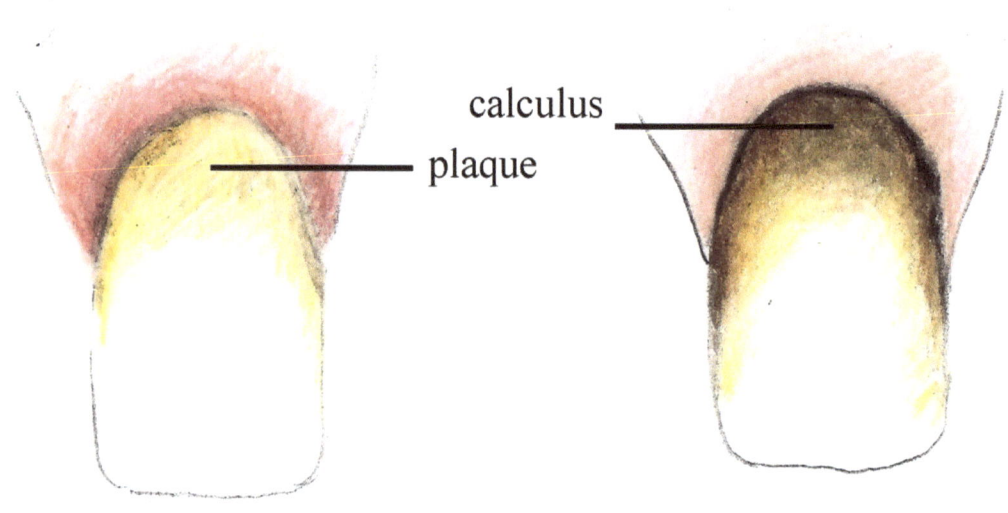

Dental Caries Process

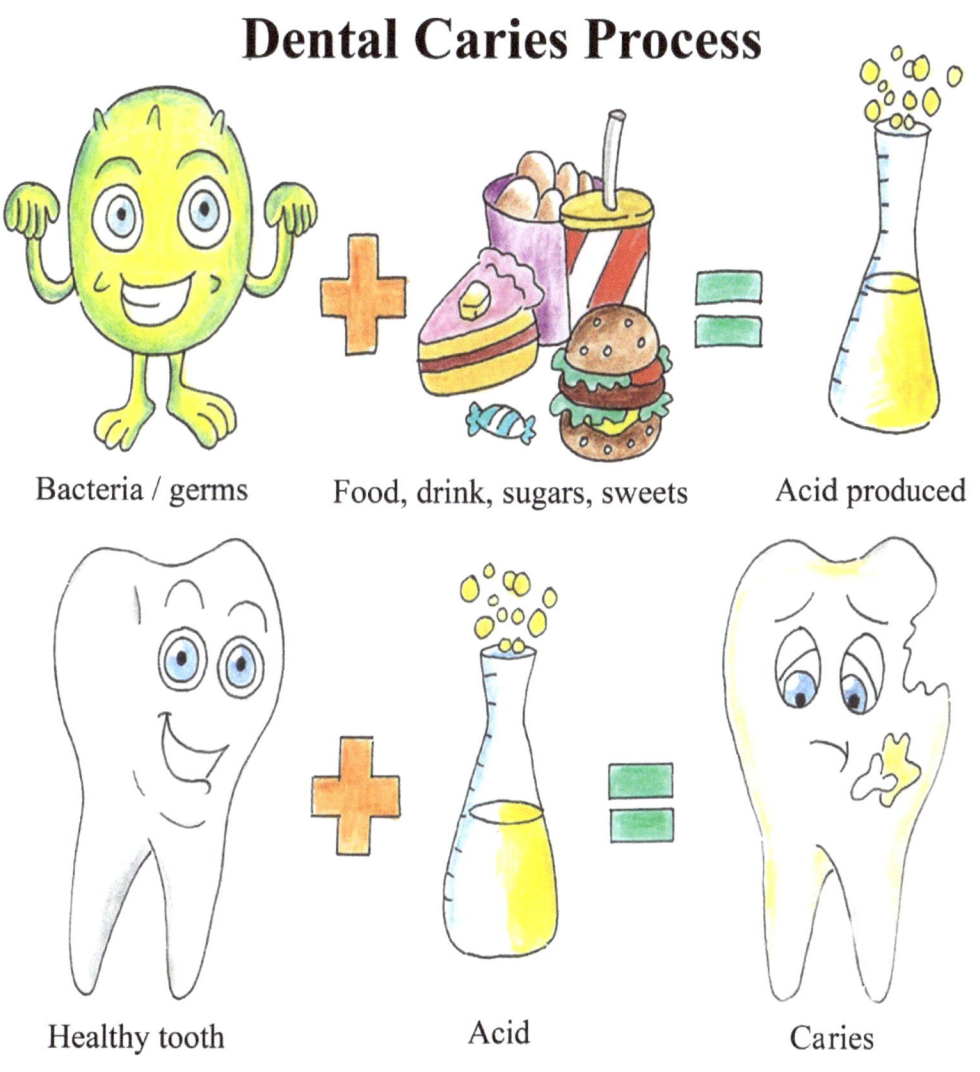

Bacteria / germs   Food, drink, sugars, sweets   Acid produced

Healthy tooth   Acid   Caries

*I*f plaque is left on the tooth for a longer time, microorganisms from plaque and food residue start to produce different acids, which begin to dissolve your tooth.

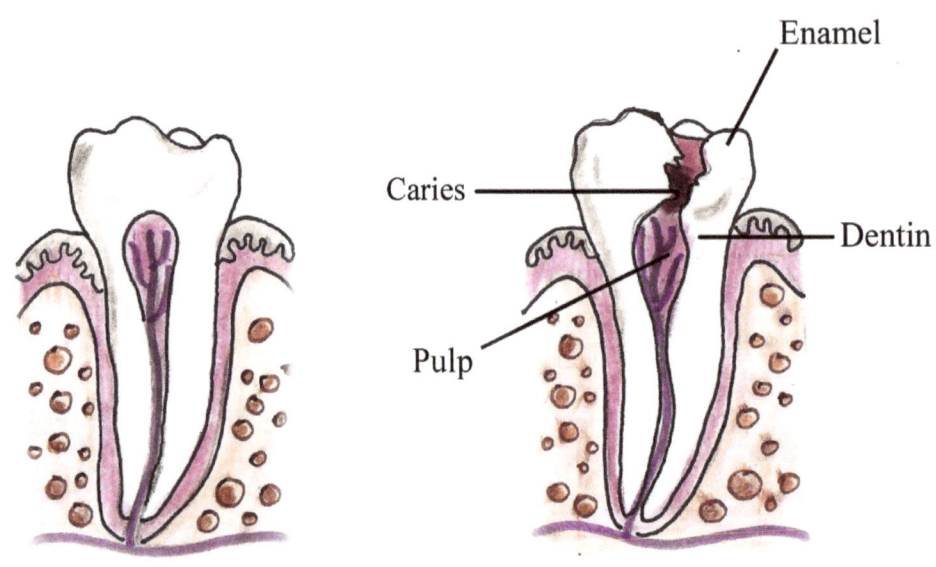

This condition is called tooth caries or tooth decay.

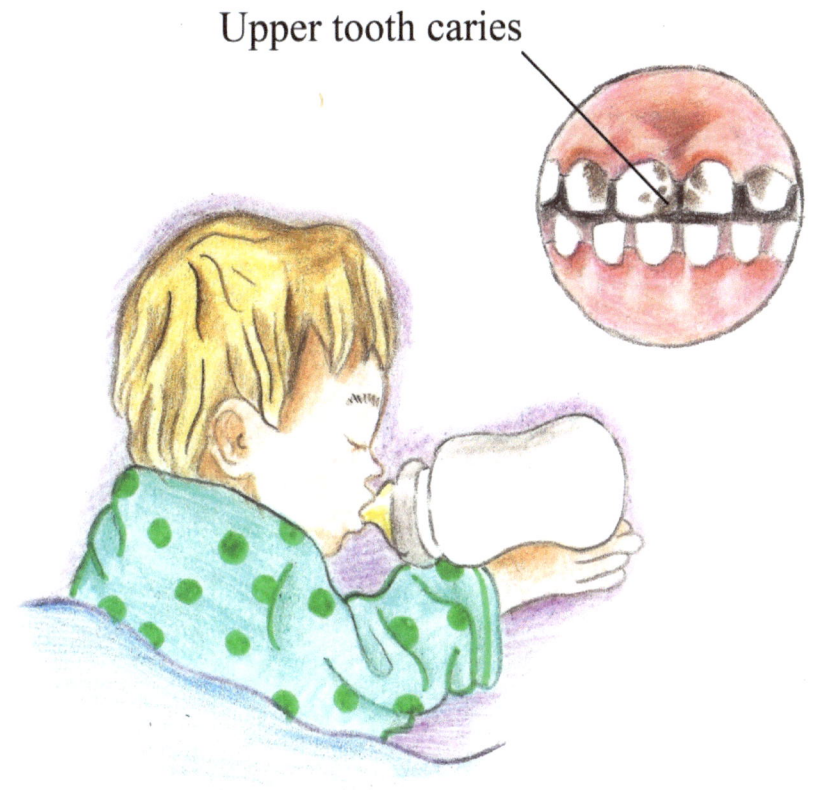

Upper tooth caries

Prolonged drinking of juice from the bottle can also cause caries, **especially in younger** children. Therefore, that should be avoided, especially before bed time.

In conclusion, if you do not **brush** your teeth properly, bacteria and microorganisms from the plaque on and around the tooth will be very active and will start to dissolve your tooth and as a result you will start to feel pain during eating or drinking. Your tooth will not look nice like a mountain with all cusps and fissures, but instead it will have a "hole".

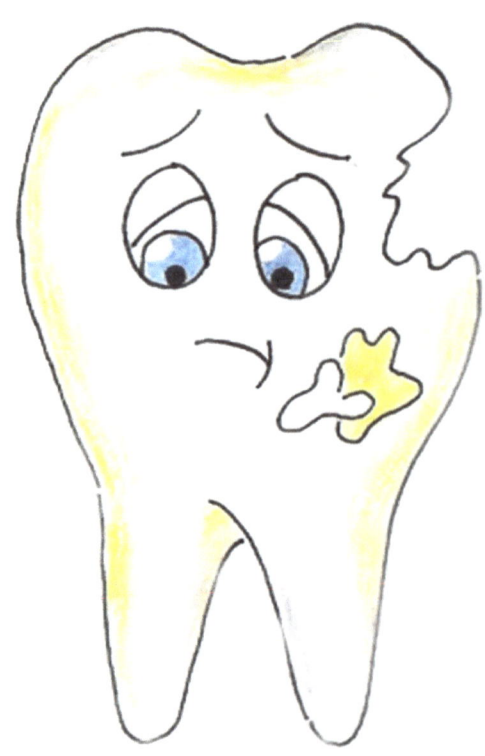

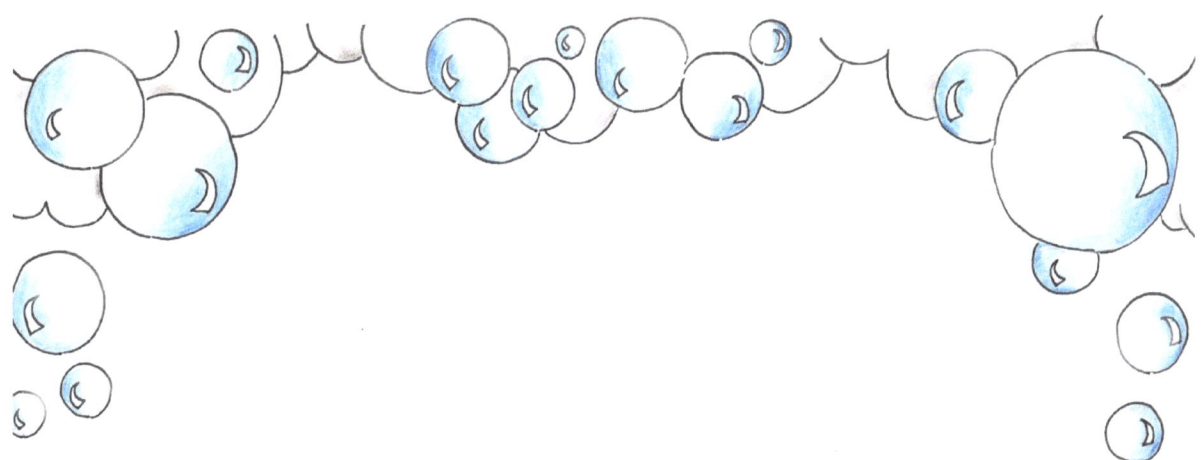

What do you do in that case?

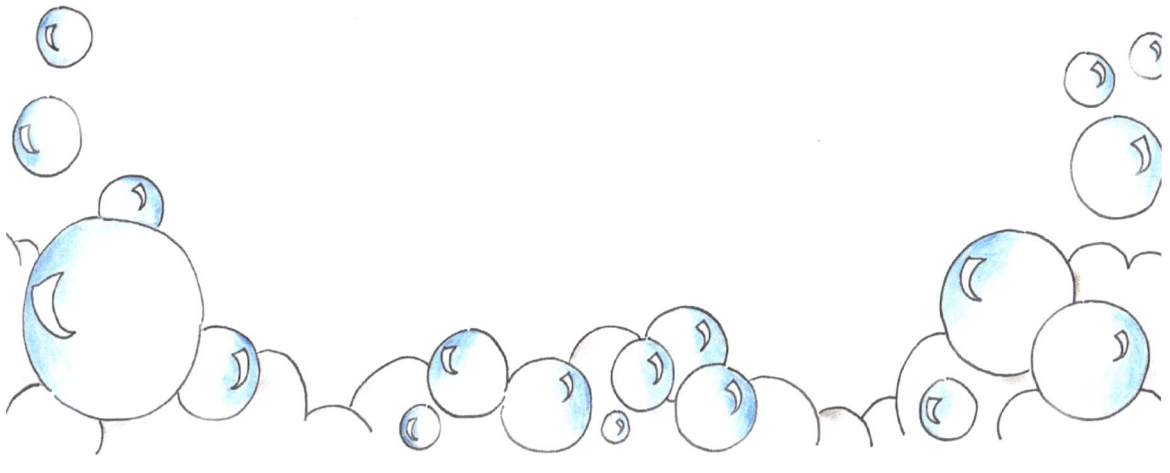

You will have to visit the dentist. The dentist will use special instruments to examine your teeth – mirror and explorer.

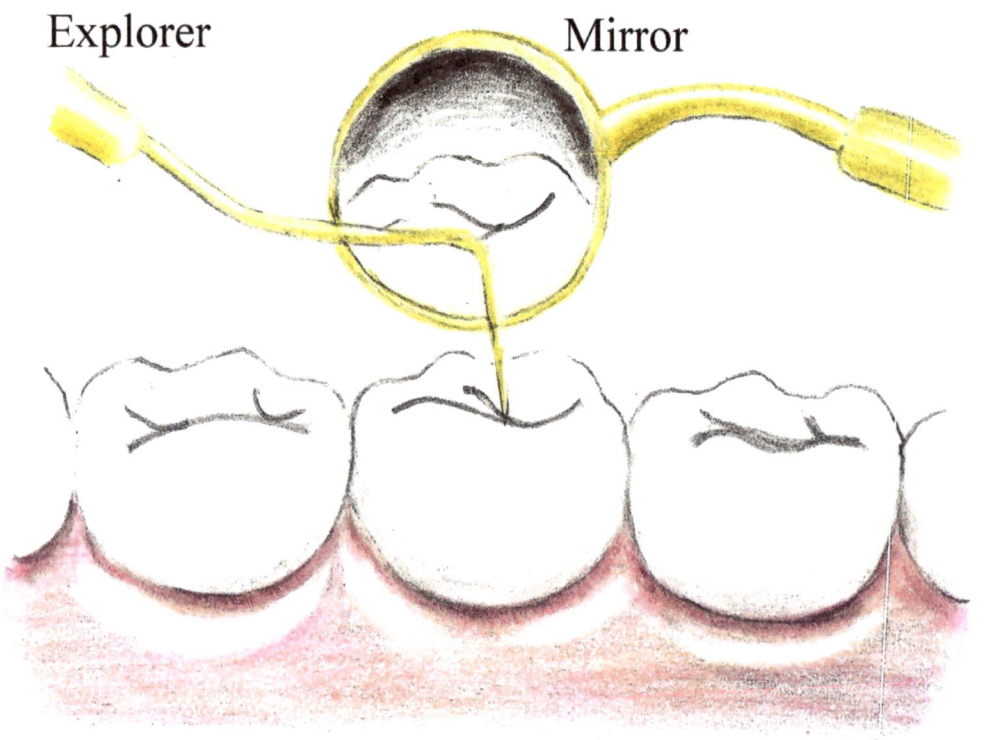

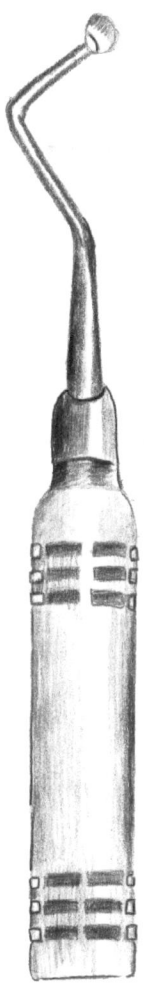

Also, the dentist will use specially designed instruments to remove all bacteria and microorganisms from your tooth, so called hand instruments, like an excavator. An excavator looks like a small spoon.

Further, the dentist will use a turbine and a micro motor – special hand **pieces (or drill)** with bur on it to additionally remove destroyed tooth substance.

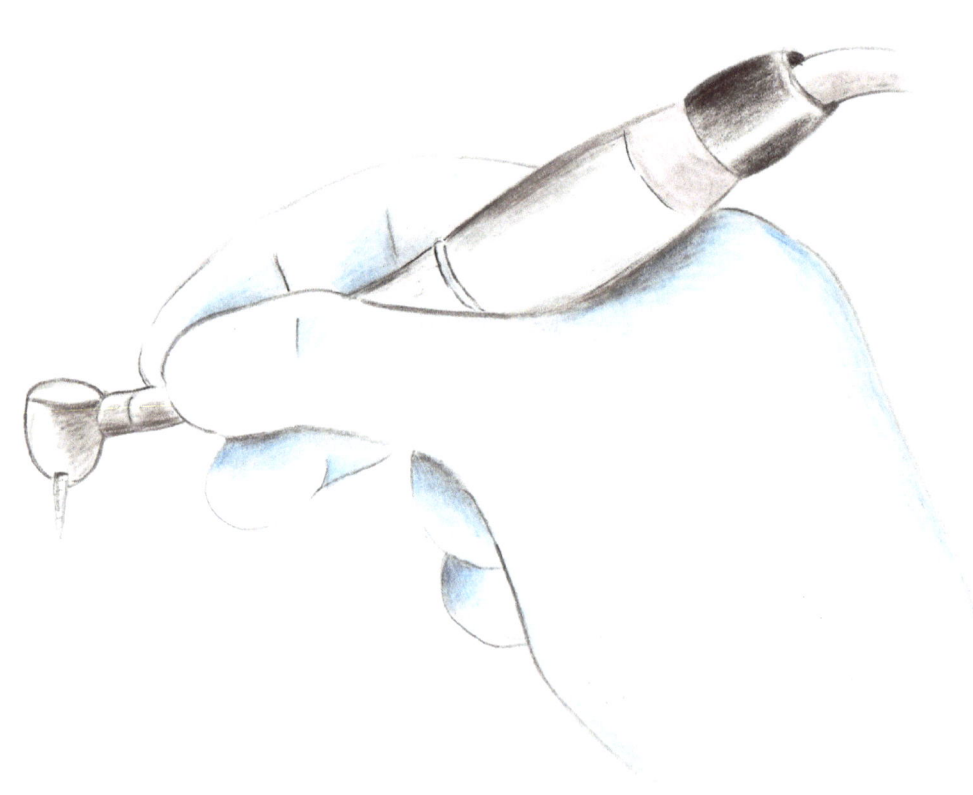

These hand-pieces sprinkle water while **working**, making them look like a shower. The water sprinkling from the hand-pieces prevents the tooth from heat which is produced during removal of caries with a hand-piece.

After the dentist opens the tooth and has cleaned the caries,

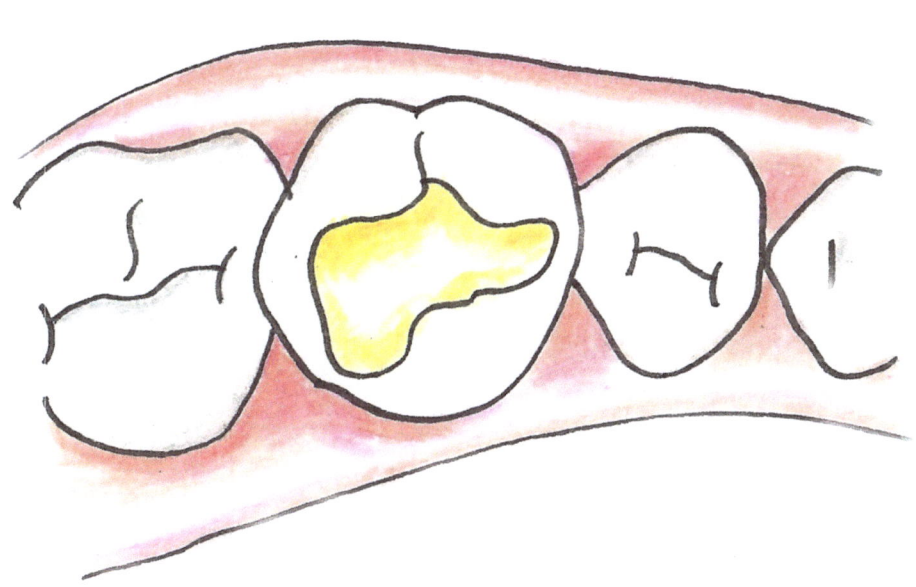

the missing tooth tissue is replaced with artificial material called amalgam

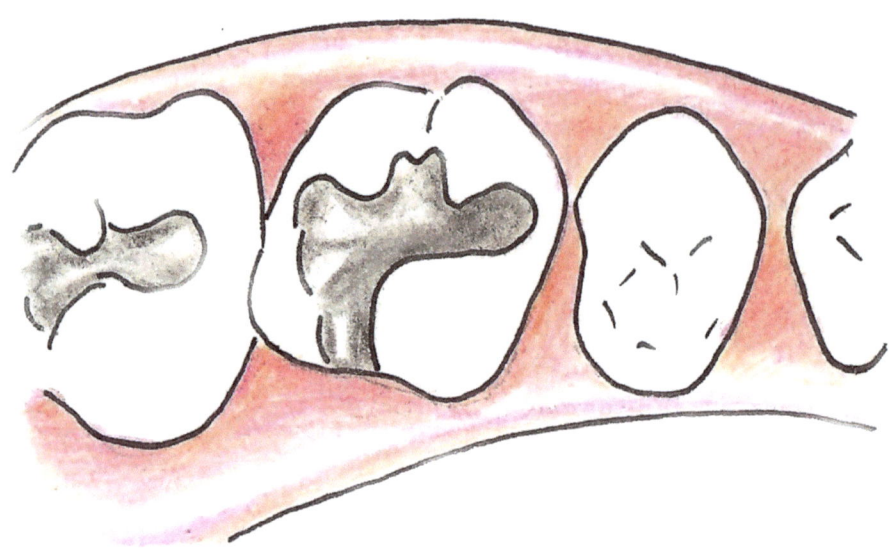

or composite material.

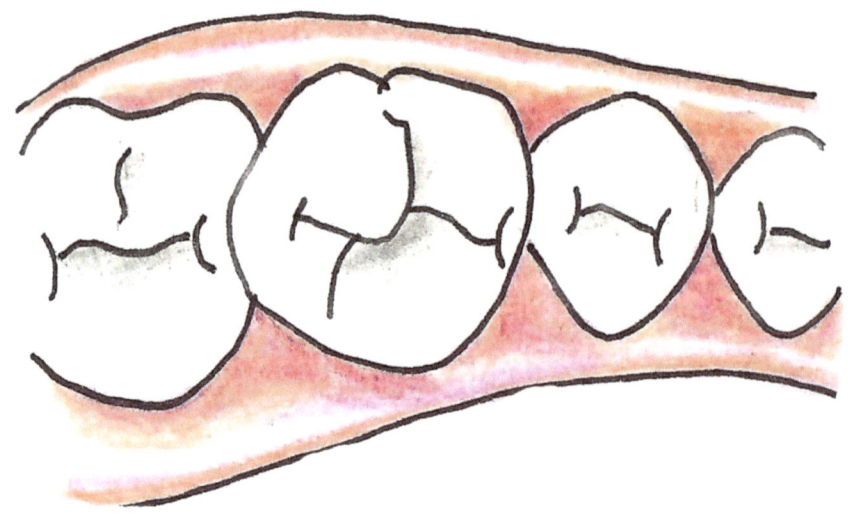

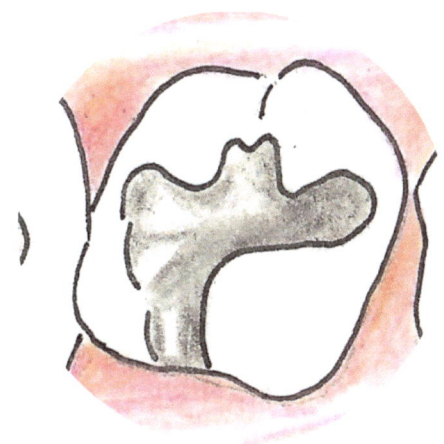

Amalgam is silver color ...

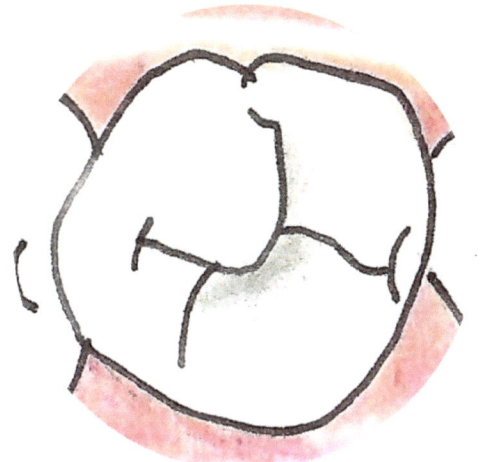

... and composite material has the same color as a healthy tooth.

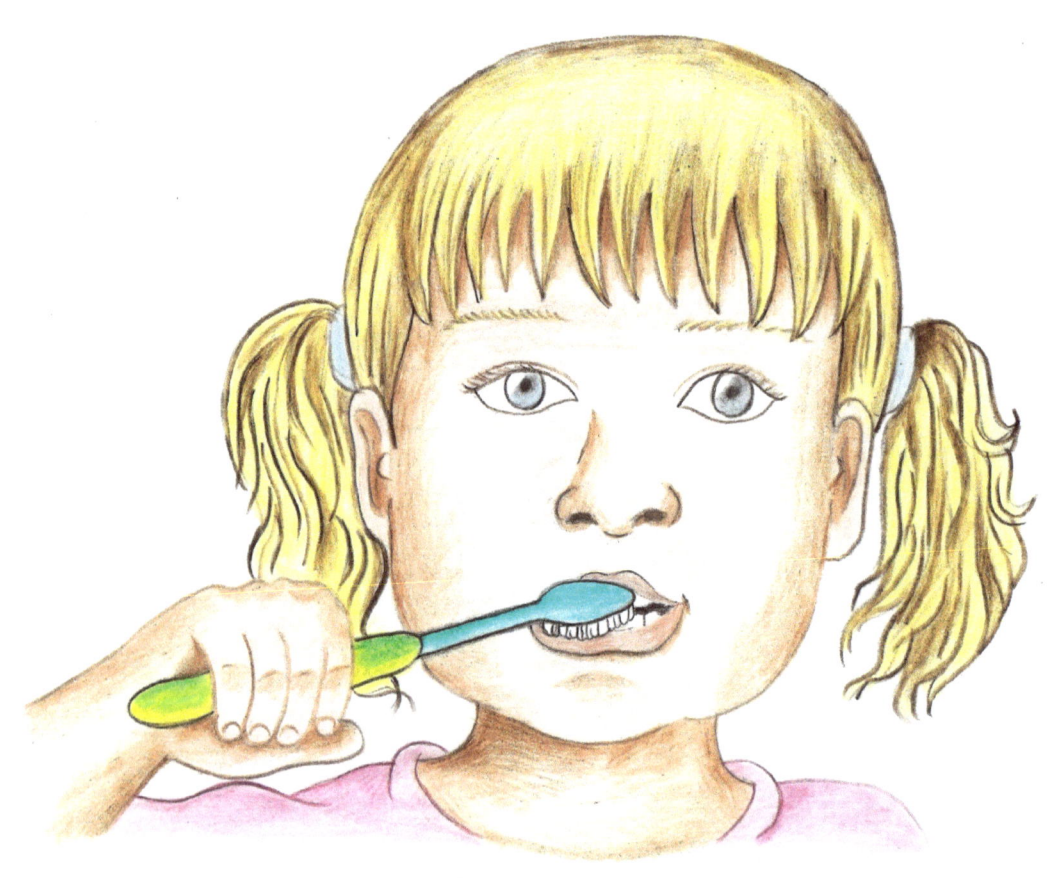

To prevent plaque accumulation and tooth caries formation, you should properly brush your teeth.

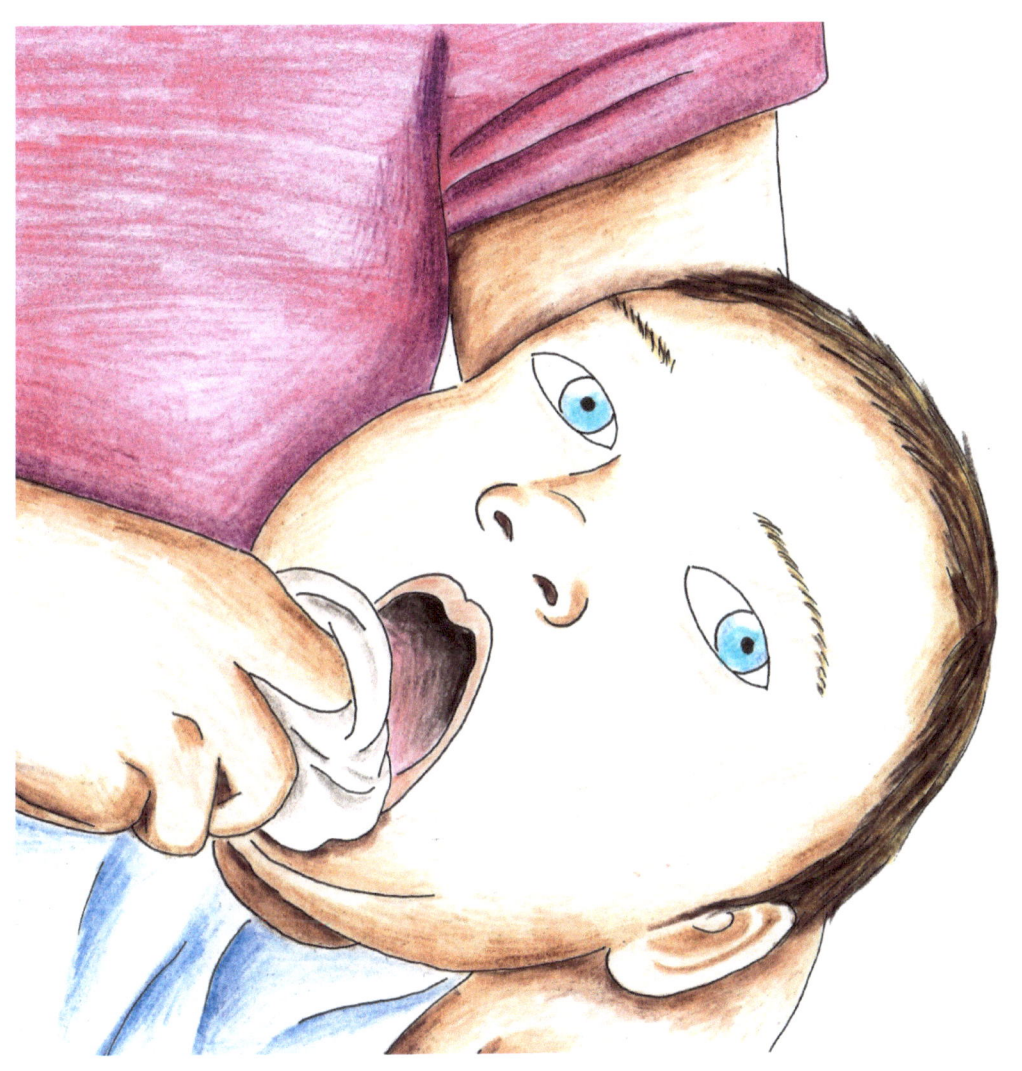

With small babies it is sometimes very difficult to brush the teeth and therefore soft cloth is used for cleaning their teeth.

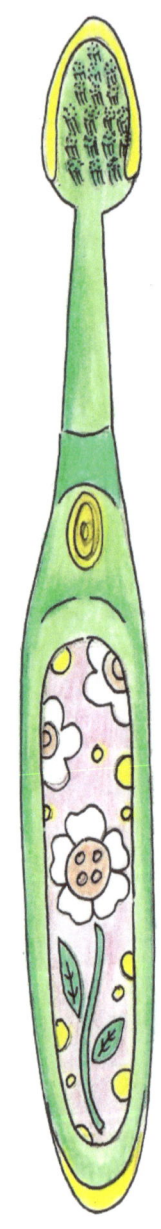

This will be enough when the baby has only front teeth, but as the baby starts getting molars, a toothbrush should be used.

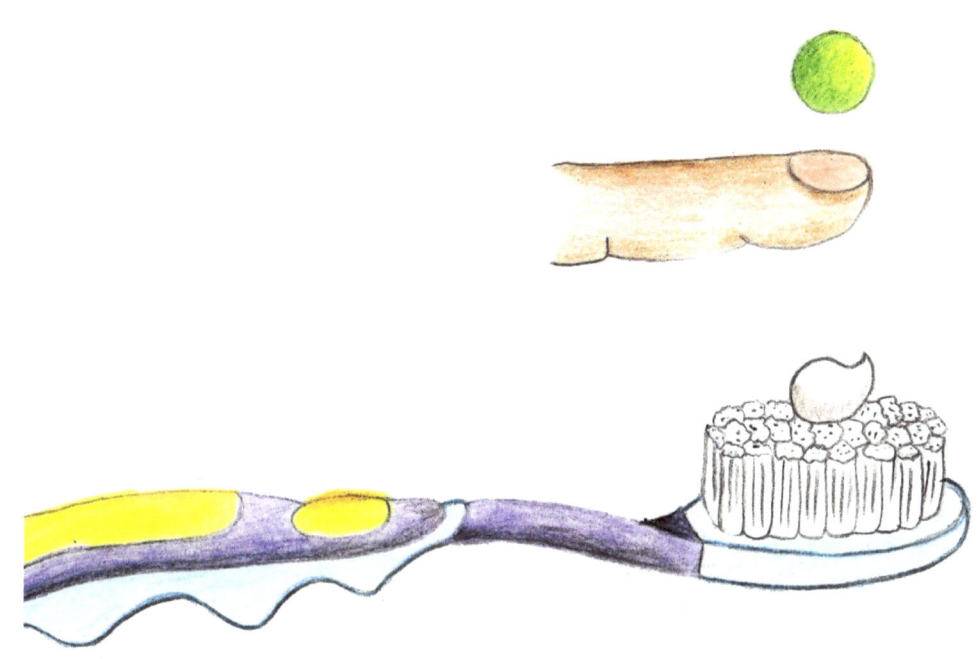

First, you will use toothbrush with water only and as you get little older you should use brush along with toothpaste. A pea size amount of paste or even less, like a size of a rice grain, will be more than enough.

Children should use toothbrushes with soft, rounded bristles for gentle cleaning. The same toothbrush should not be used longer than three months.

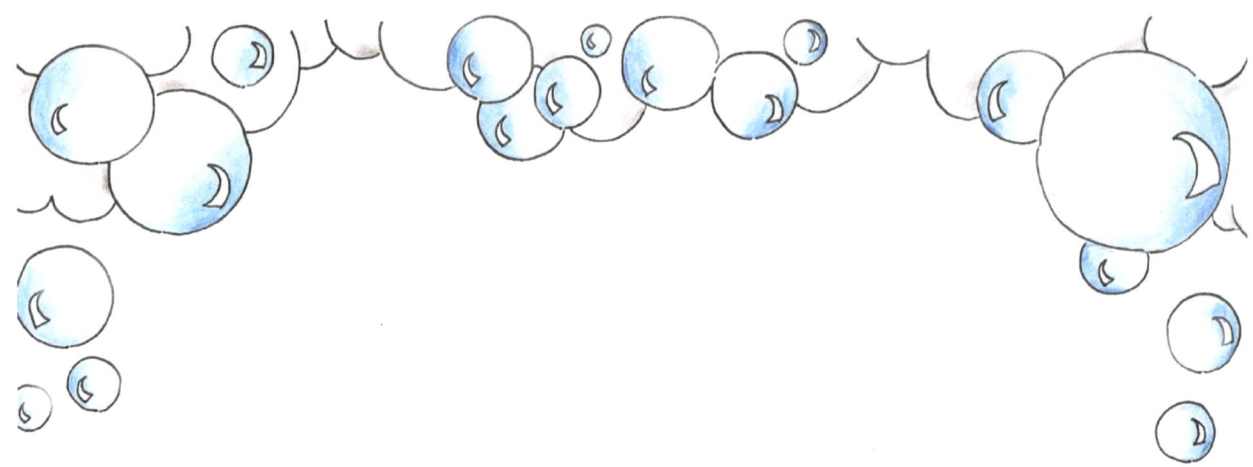

How to brush the teeth?

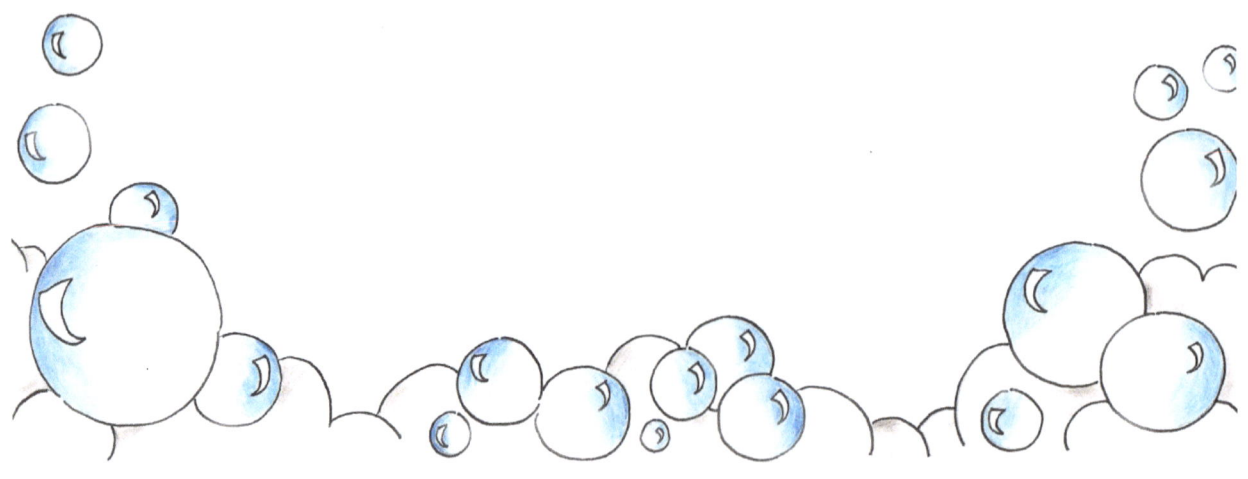

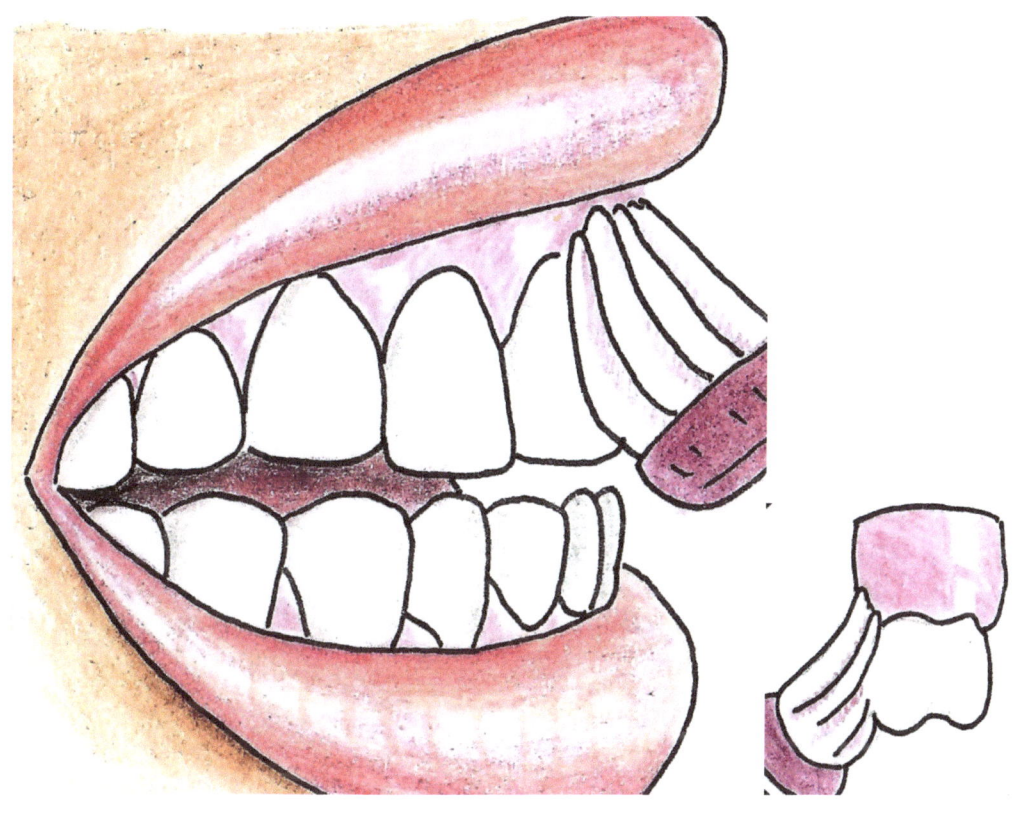

Put a pea size amount of a toothpaste on a dry brush. Place the toothbrush bristles along the gingival margin (gumline) at 45°.
The toothbrush bristles should contact the tooth surface and the gingival margin at the same time.

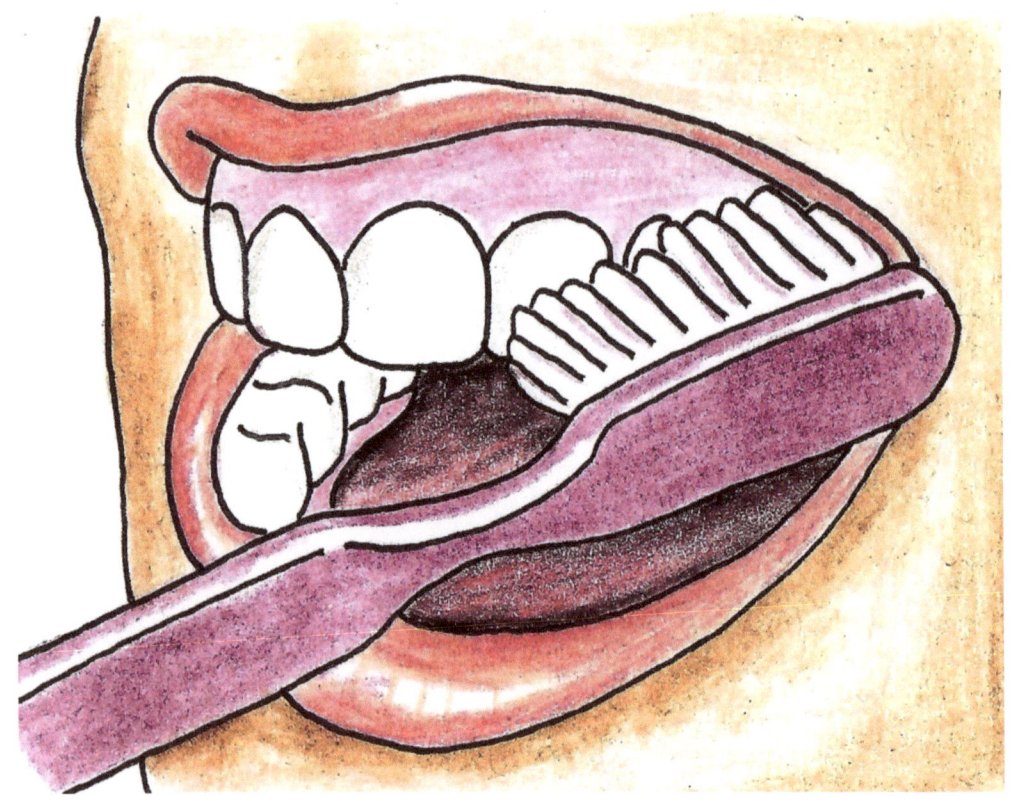

First, brush the outer tooth surface of each tooth very gently with rolling motion. Always start from one side, upper or lower, left or right and brush one by one tooth. Make sure not to skip any.

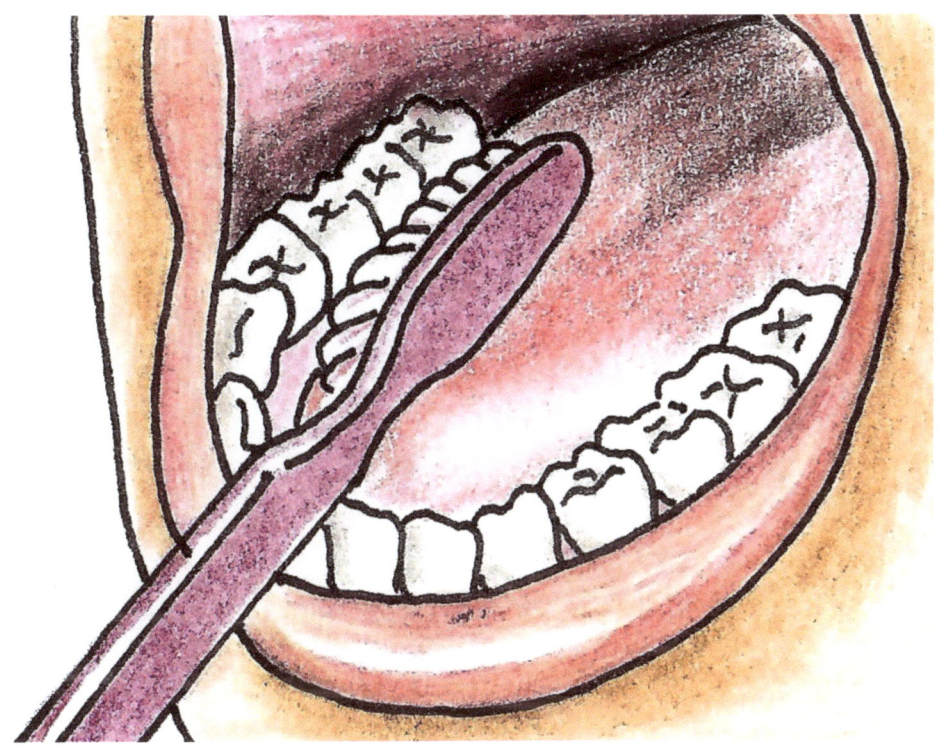

Then, place the **toothbrush bristles** in the same manner as when brushing outer surfaces. Again, start from one side, upper or lower, left or right and gently brush the inner surfaces of each tooth with rolling motion.

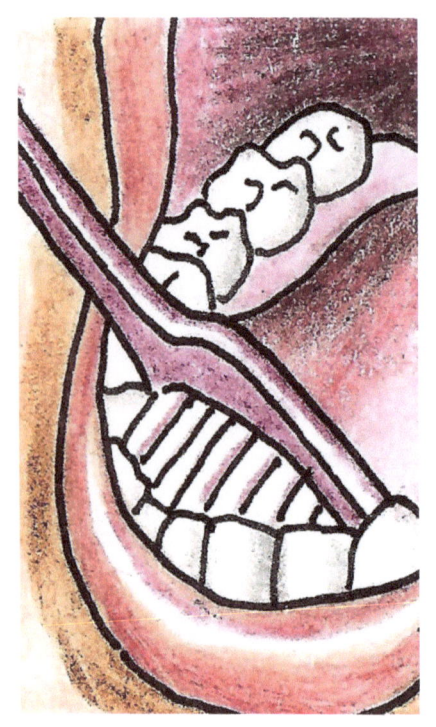 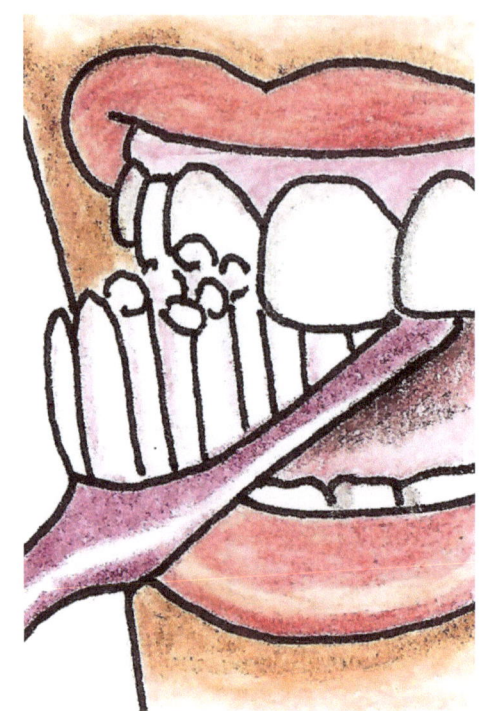

After you finished cleaning outer and inner tooth surfaces, tilt the toothbrush vertically behind the front teeth and brush with an up and down motion.

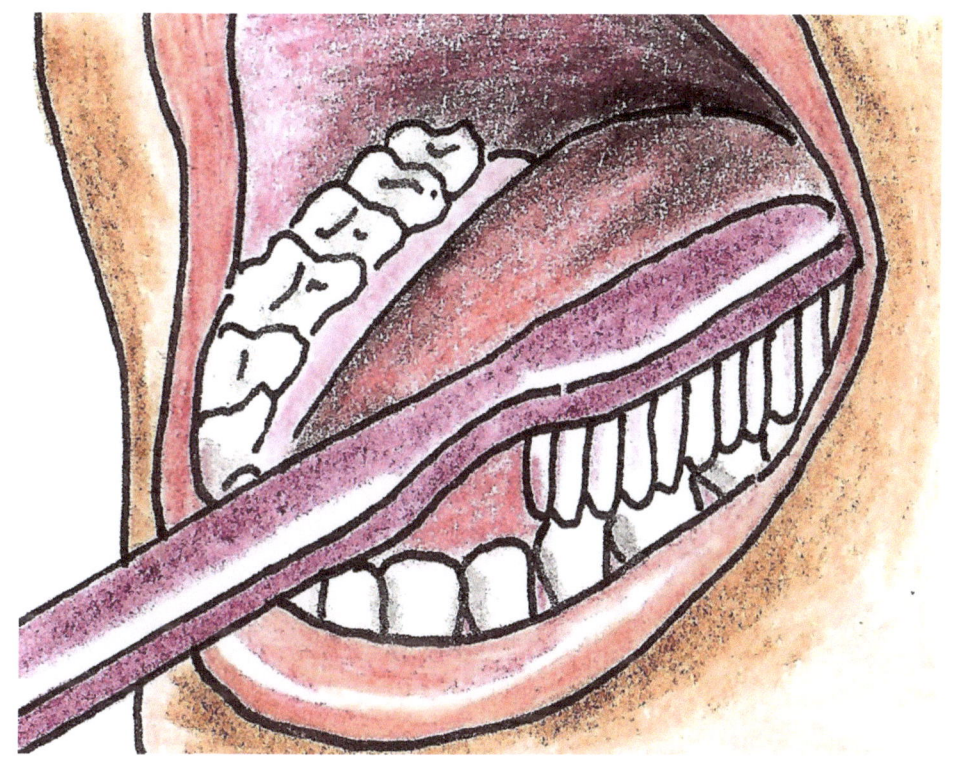

At the end, place the toothbrush against the chewing surfaces of the teeth and use a back and forth motion.

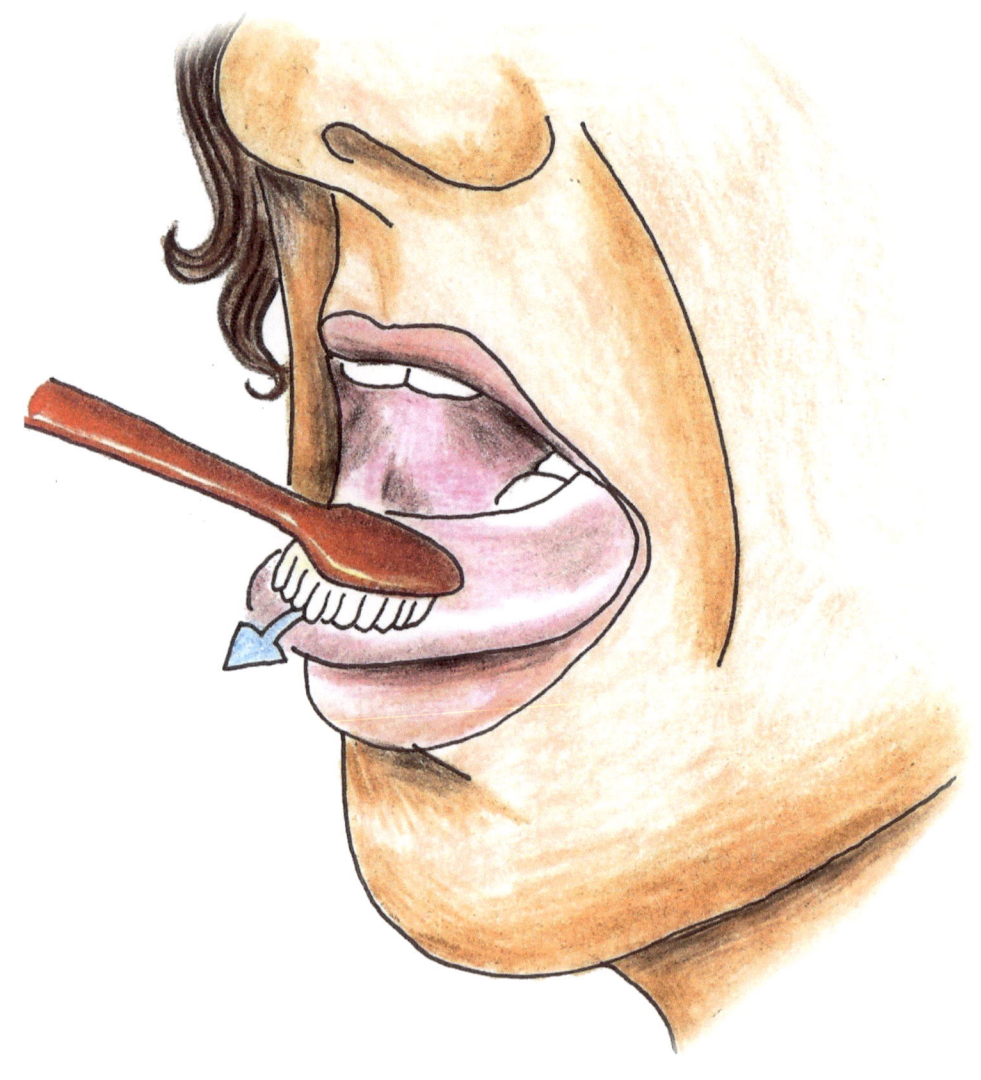

The tongue has to be cleaned as well. Gently brush the tongue to remove debris and odor-producing bacteria.

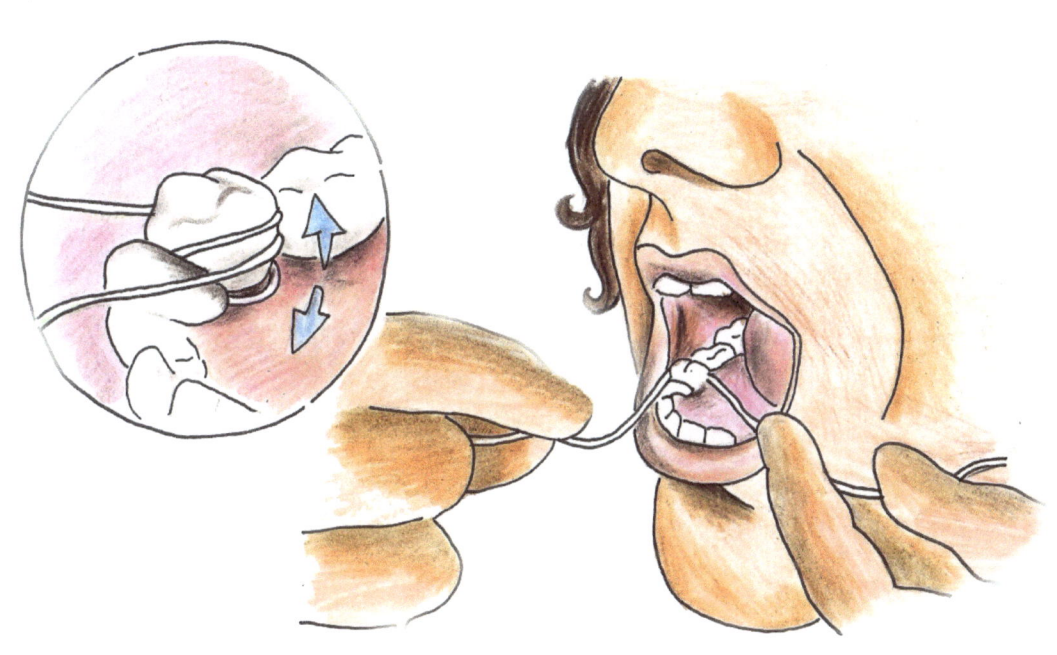

Floss **between the teeth** daily. This way you are cleaning interdental area, spaces between each tooth, which cannot be cleaned very well with the toothbrush.

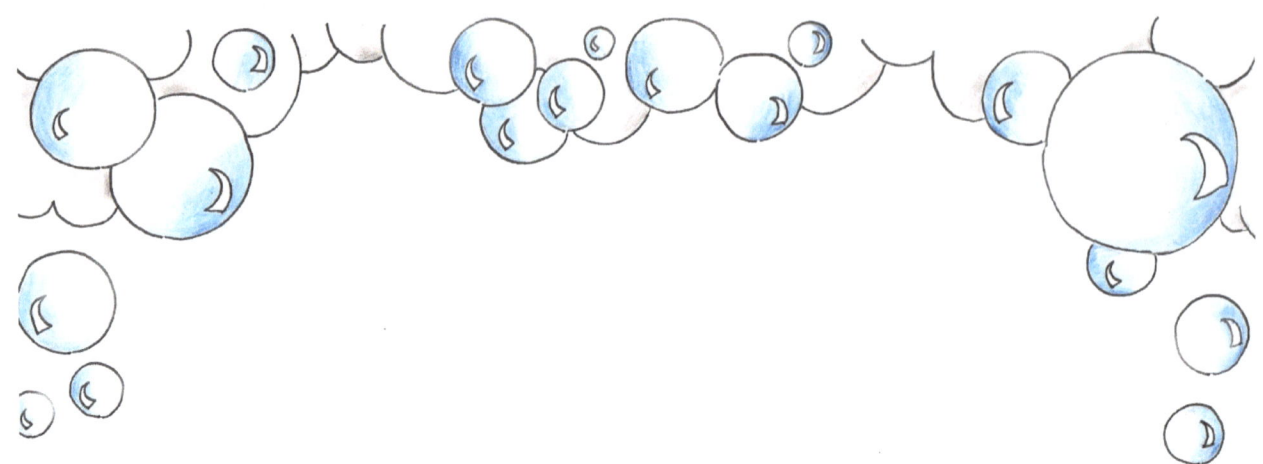

Of course, do not forget to visit your dentist regularly!

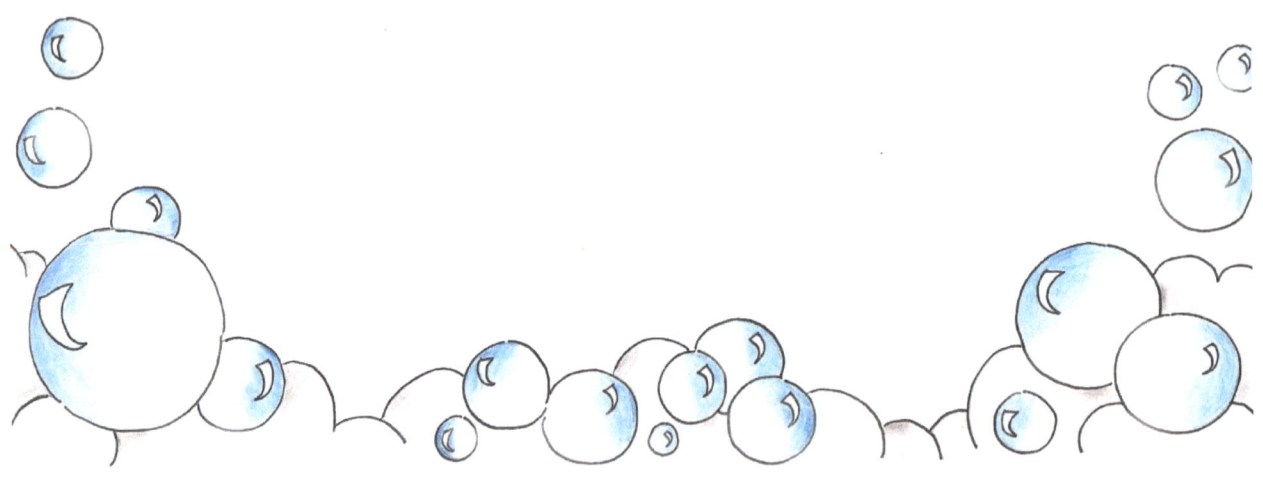

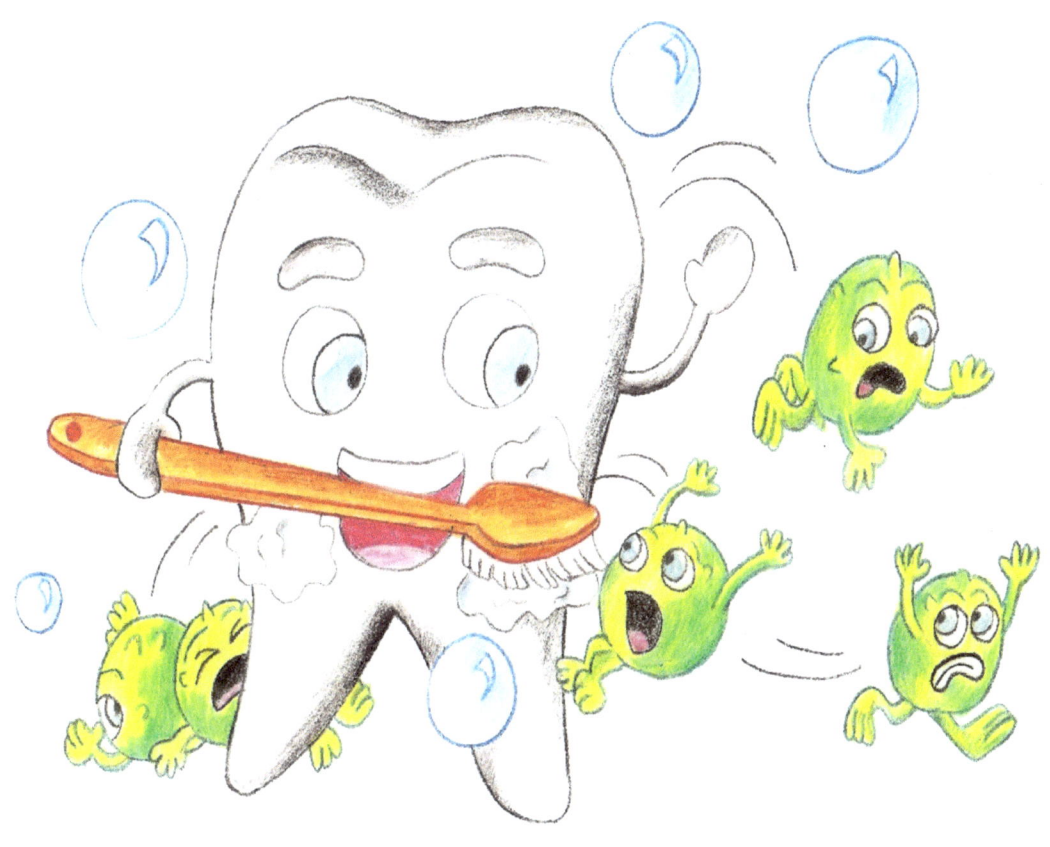

By doing so, your teeth will be healthy and happy and you will be happy as well!!!

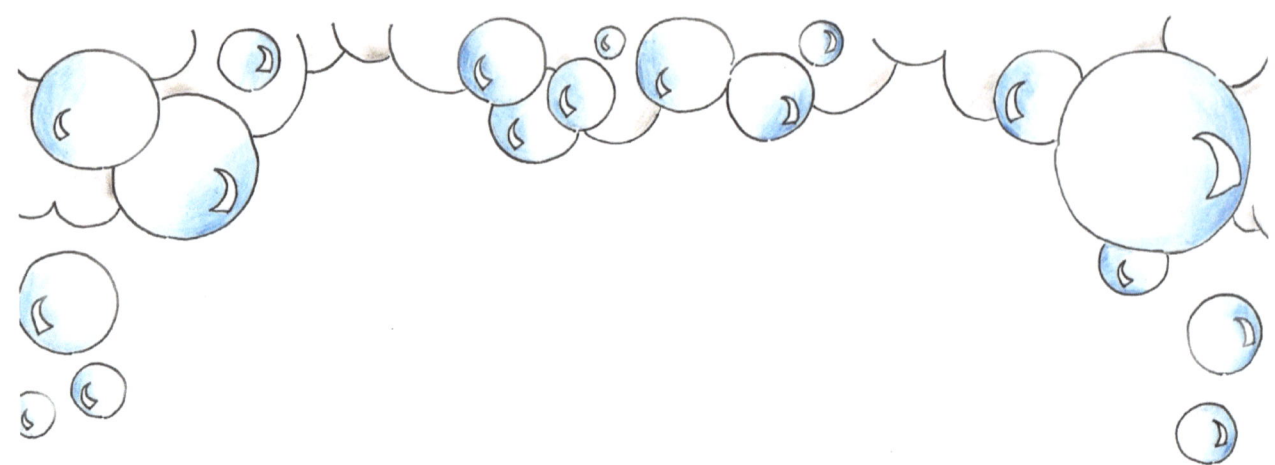

Appendix

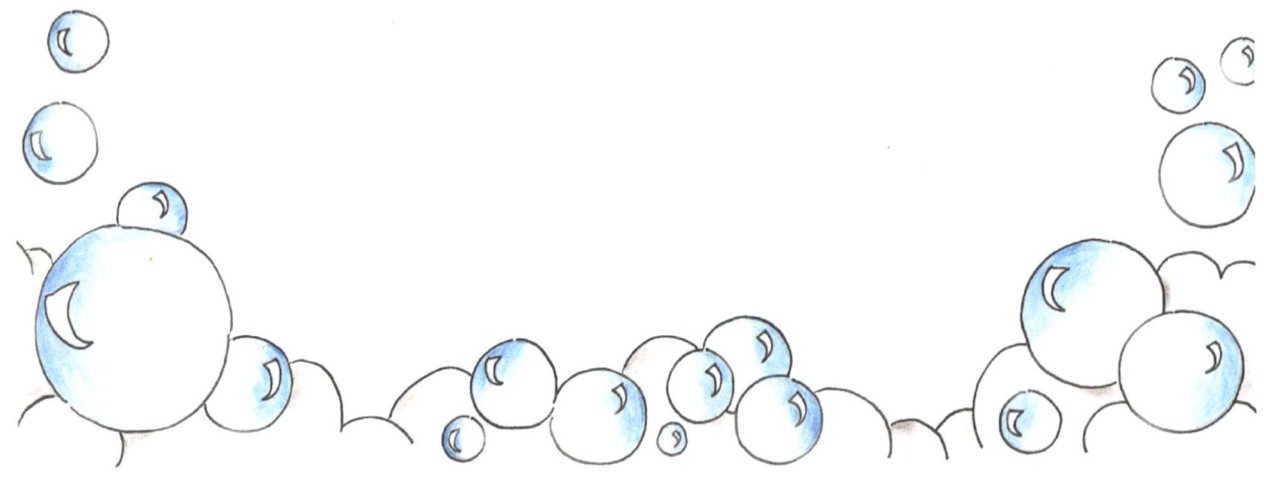

*T*ips for parents:

- ✓ Help your children to follow a healthy diet.
- ✓ Help your children to establish good dental care habits.
- ✓ Help your children to brush their teeth at least twice a day using a soft-bristled brush, for at least two minutes.
- ✓ Help them until they can do a good job themselves, at least until age 7, 8, or even 9. Even thereafter you should check if they have done their job properly.
- ✓ Help them to floss their teeth before bedtime.
- ✓ Visit your dentist regularly.
- ✓ Watch for signs of any unusual behavior of your child and talk to your dentist if you see any warning signs such as: sucking on cheeks, sucking on lips, problems with chewing food, problems with sleeping, reluctance to smile, aching teeth or gingiva.

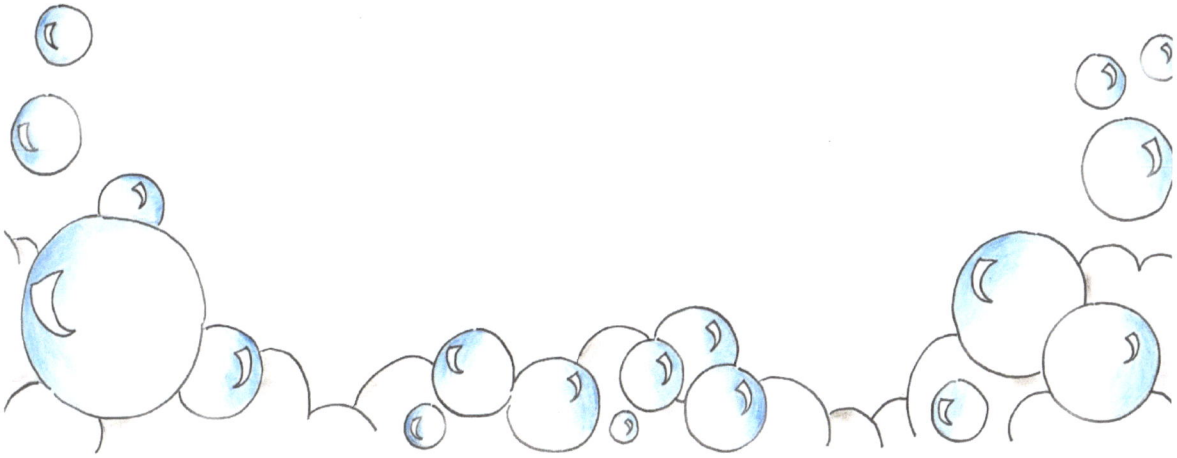

- ✓ When your child **starts to get permanent teeth (beginning with six years of** age) talk to you dentist about sealants.
- ✓ Sealants can be applied to the fissures of the chewing surfaces of teeth in order to prevent plaque accumulation and caries formation. With the **sealants, teeth** cleaning will **be** much easier.
- ✓ Sealants should be applied as soon as the tooth appears in the oral cavity.

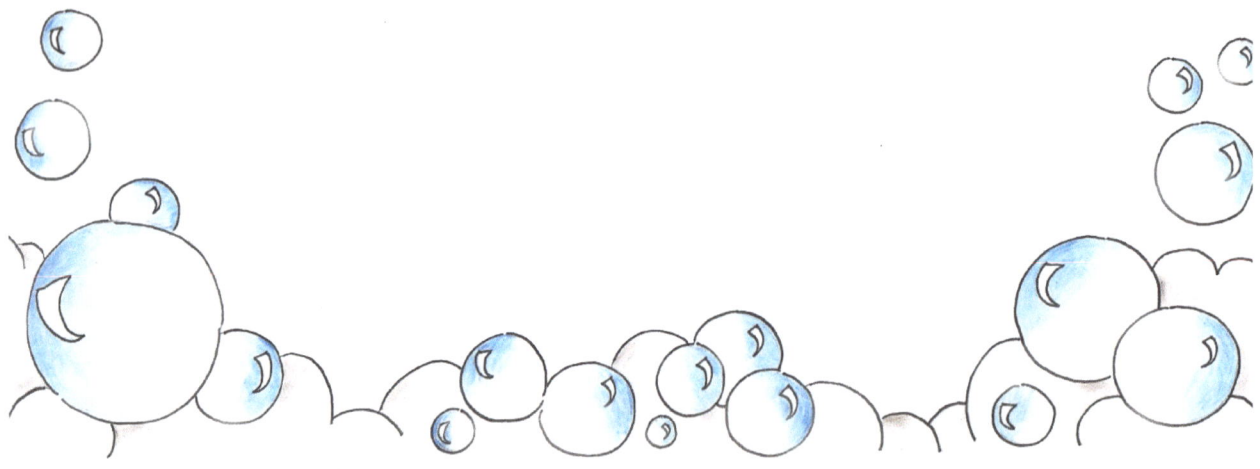

Primary/Deciduous dentition (baby teeth)

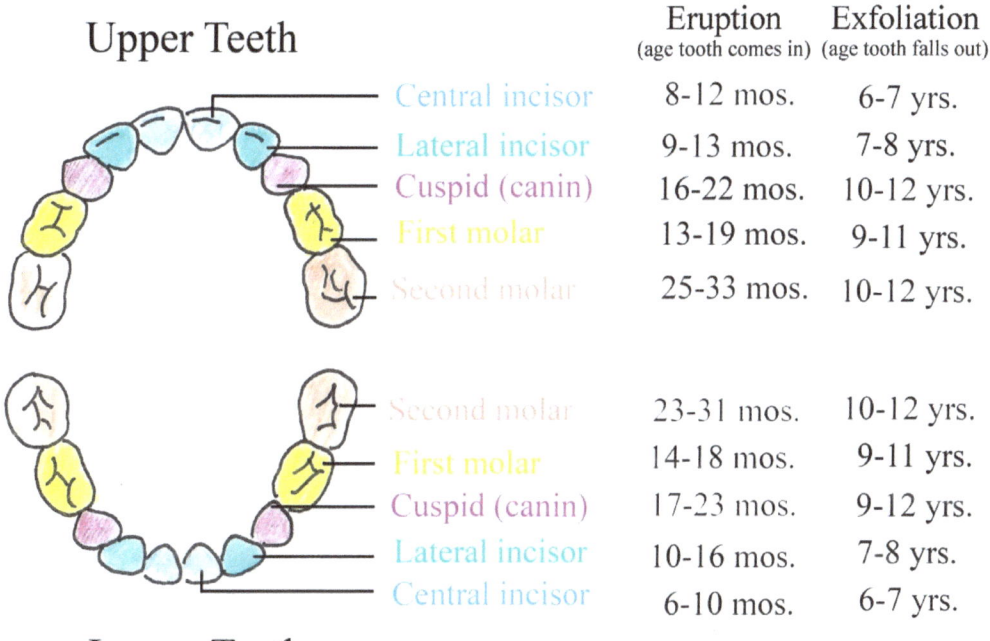

Upper Teeth	Eruption (age tooth comes in)	Exfoliation (age tooth falls out)
Central incisor	8-12 mos.	6-7 yrs.
Lateral incisor	9-13 mos.	7-8 yrs.
Cuspid (canin)	16-22 mos.	10-12 yrs.
First molar	13-19 mos.	9-11 yrs.
Second molar	25-33 mos.	10-12 yrs.

Lower Teeth	Eruption	Exfoliation
Second molar	23-31 mos.	10-12 yrs.
First molar	14-18 mos.	9-11 yrs.
Cuspid (canin)	17-23 mos.	9-12 yrs.
Lateral incisor	10-16 mos.	7-8 yrs.
Central incisor	6-10 mos.	6-7 yrs.

Permanent dentition (adult teeth)

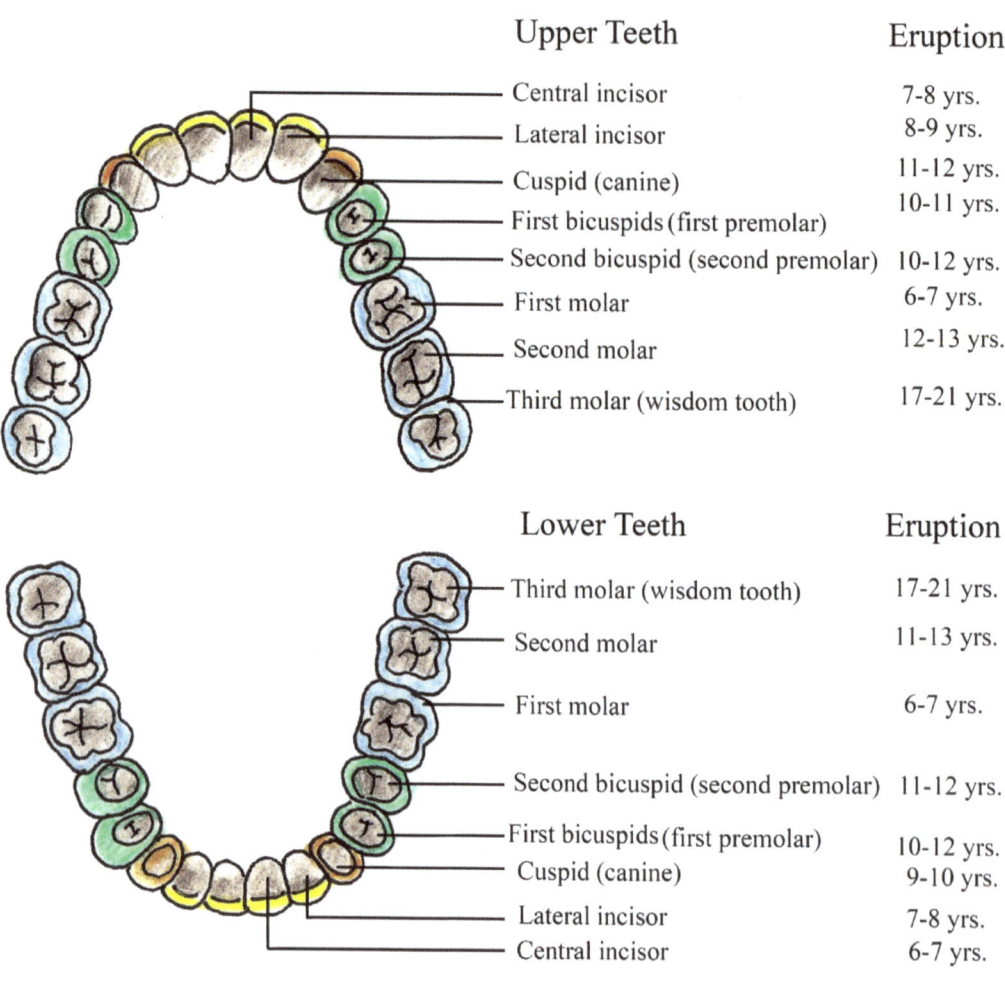

Upper Teeth	Eruption
Central incisor	7-8 yrs.
Lateral incisor	8-9 yrs.
Cuspid (canine)	11-12 yrs.
First bicuspids (first premolar)	10-11 yrs.
Second bicuspid (second premolar)	10-12 yrs.
First molar	6-7 yrs.
Second molar	12-13 yrs.
Third molar (wisdom tooth)	17-21 yrs.

Lower Teeth	Eruption
Third molar (wisdom tooth)	17-21 yrs.
Second molar	11-13 yrs.
First molar	6-7 yrs.
Second bicuspid (second premolar)	11-12 yrs.
First bicuspids (first premolar)	10-12 yrs.
Cuspid (canine)	9-10 yrs.
Lateral incisor	7-8 yrs.
Central incisor	6-7 yrs.

For my memories...

I got my first tooth when I was _____ months old.

When I visit the dentist for the first time I was _____ months/years old.

I lost my first tooth when I was _____ years old and got my first permanent tooth when I was_____years old.

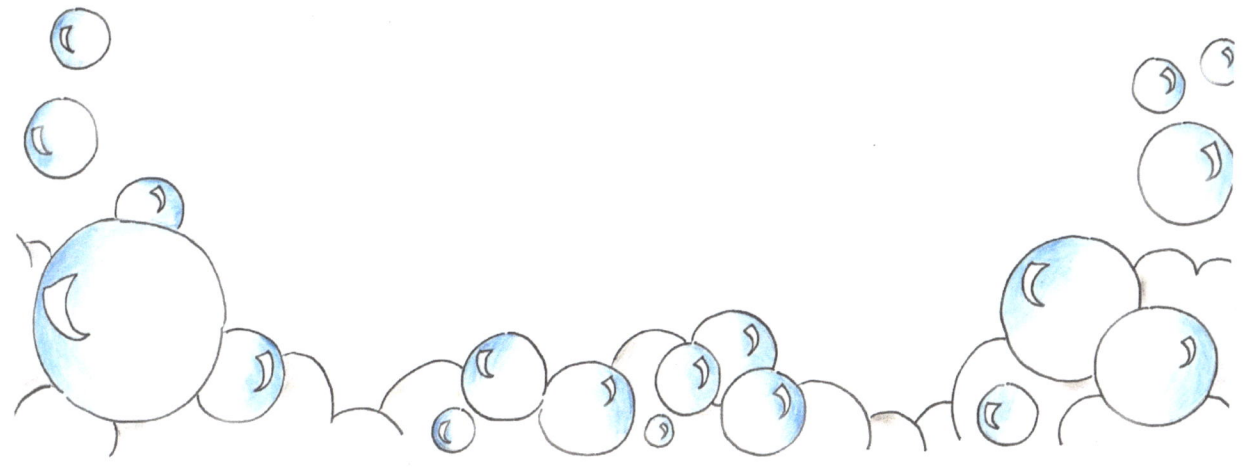

BRUSH-TRASH-FLASH SONG

I got a new, new, brush
*A*nd I put the box in the trash, trash, trash,
*T*hen I put a paste a size of rice on my brand new brush
*A*nd I start to clean my teeth doing brush, brush, brush,
*A*nd I send all bacteria in a trash, trash, trash,
*A*nd my teeth are now shining flash, flash, flash!
I will do every day brush, brush, brush,
*W*ith my brand new brush, brush, brush!

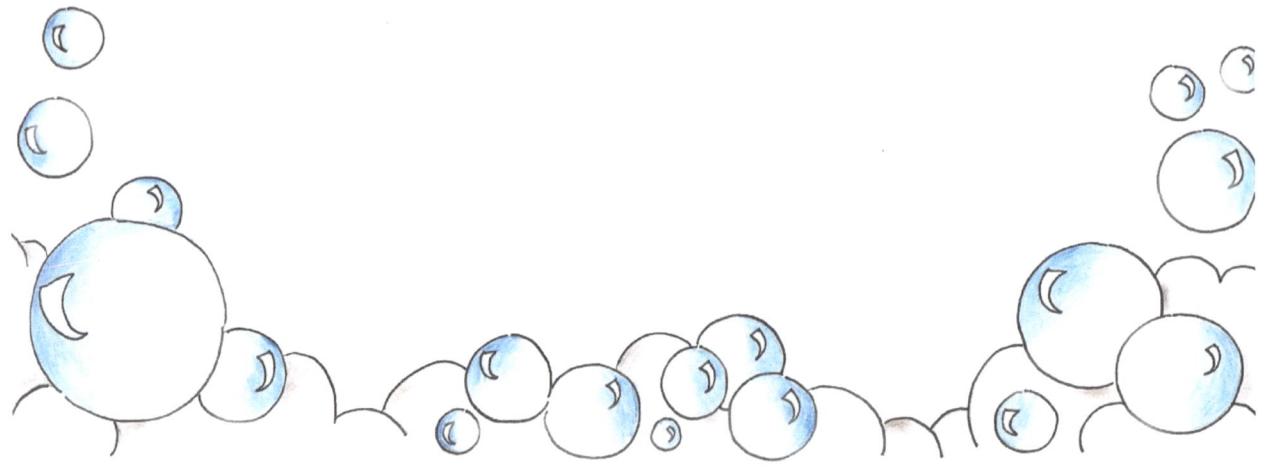

Bibliography

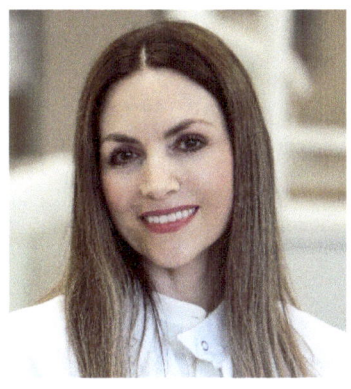

Alena Knezevic, DMD, MS, PhD, graduated from the School of Dental Medicine, University of Zagreb, Croatia, where she got her MS and PhD degree. She completed her residency program and got certified in Endodontics and Restorative Dentistry. She was a collaborator on several dental projects and grants; is the author and co-author of over 100 scientific and clinical papers and has actively participated in numerous international meetings. She was awarded with several awards for the research in the field or composite materials, curing lights and photopolymerization. She completed postdoc program at the Ludwig Maximillian University in Munich, Germany. She works as a Clinical Assistant Professor at the Herman Ostrow School of Dentistry, University of Southern California, Los Angeles, where she teaches Operative Dentistry and CAD/CAM. She is also a Croatian language teacher at the St. Anthony Croatian Childrens' School and is the author of several childrens' picture books.

Photo by John Skalicky

www.ingramcontent.com/pod-product-compliance
Lightning Source LLC
Chambersburg PA
CBHW051208220526
45473CB00003B/948